For my grandchildren,

Kyriacos, Alexander, Gabriel, Nico

and Daisy,

to inspire them to explore the wonderful
countryside of Britain.

Afoot and light-hearted I take to the open road,

Healthy, free, the world before me.

The long brown path before me leading wherever I choose.

.....will you come travel with me?

From Song of the Open Road by Walt Whitman

Acknowledgements

I would like to thank Ian for joining me when he could and helping and supporting me throughout the walk and the writing of this book. It would have been difficult to achieve the challenge without his love and guidance.

I am truly grateful for the friends who walked with me: Dawn, Avril, Linda, Jacky, Carole, Glennys and Andrew, Scottish Sue and Cleethorpes Sue. Their chat and laughter cheered me immensely.

My family were also stalwart supporters. Nick and Kat walked with me as did Tim, Chris, Andy, Jenny and Isla. I was also joined by Rachel, Jorge and Chenoa. Wonderful memories! Special thanks to Patsy for supporting me with her camper van and looking after me for three weeks.

I would like to thank Lorraine Anderson for her patient proofreading.

Thanks also to Dawn and Patsy for the loan of some maps. I'd like to thank Chris Griffin and family for a wonderful and much needed two days of rest and recuperation at their house. Also to Glennys and Andrew for a comfortable overnight stay with them which included an evening tour of the historical highlights of Lichfield.

A big thank you to all my friends and family who were unable to join me but kept me sane with their texts and phone calls.

Lastly I would like to thank Sue Campbell who inspired me to raise money on my walk for the "Drive for Grimsby" Fund which helps disadvantaged youngsters of North East Lincolnshire take part in the activities of the Duke of Edinburgh Award Scheme. Thanks to all who donated to the total of £3000.

Contents

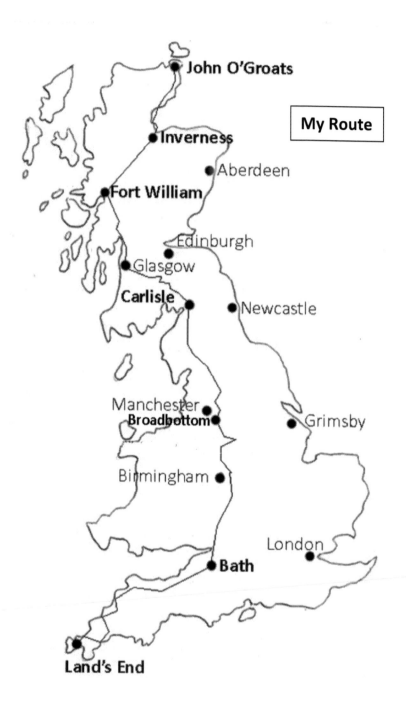

My Route

John O'Groats

Inverness

Aberdeen

Fort William

Edinburgh

Glasgow

Carlisle

Newcastle

Manchester

Broadbottom

Grimsby

Birmingham

London

Bath

Land's End

Introduction

Adventure after Cancer

My walk from Land's End to John O'Groats

It was a scary distance. I wondered if I could make it. I felt like a very old person as I tentatively put one foot in front of the other and looked for something to hang onto. It was my first attempt to try to walk from my hospital bed to the ward door after my operation.

It all happened three years ago in 2014 after I'd done one of the regular screenings that come through the post giving you the opportunity to check if you have a bowel problem. I did the simple test and sent it off. After a week or so I found out that there was something not quite right and was asked to go for a colonoscopy at the local hospital. My partner, Ian, was with me when they told us both that I had a 5cm tumour in my colon which would have to be removed. We were both in shock. I had none of the risk factors associated with bowel cancer. I've always been pretty healthy, being careful not to eat too much meat, (I eat mostly vegetarian food). I don't drink too much alcohol and I've never smoked. I exercise regularly, mostly walking but also yoga and swimming. Despite that, the reality was, I had cancer. I had a successful operation to remove part of my colon and was very lucky not to have to have a stoma bag or to need chemotherapy as the cancer had not spread. However, after nine days I got an infection and had to return to hospital for another three weeks where I was starved and pumped with antibiotics to get rid of the infection. It was an awful time. When at last I started to recover and was able to walk about, I would go exploring down the corridors. Eventually I discovered the chapel which had a piano. Ian brought me my music and I enjoyed playing that very much. Ian was a great comfort to me as he visited every day and played his guitar to me. The staff on duty would try to pop in to hear him play if they were nearby. He is a wonderful classical guitarist.

Music and walking are my great passions. I'm a music teacher and have taught many pupils in schools all over Grimsby and Cleethorpes and many private pupils at home too. I play the piano, classical guitar and flute. I love playing in ensembles with friends and also accompany a choir, the Waltham Choral Society. I enjoy playing flute in the Grimsby Symphony Orchestra too. So you see when I couldn't walk and was so ill it focussed me on how short life is. (I'm 69 now). I realised that if there's anything you want to do in life you must do it now. I was told that if I hadn't done the screening test and the cancer hadn't been spotted I would have been dead in four years.

I've not always loved walking. When I was a child I was taken on walking holidays with my parents, often to Derbyshire or Yorkshire and I *did* enjoy them. That was my introduction to walking and I think that memory was instilled into my brain of loving being in the countryside. However, as a teenager, my older sister, Patsy, called me "a townie" as I said I hated walking and didn't want to go out in the countryside, or go on family holidays. I remember being made to go to a farm with my parents when I was sixteen. I was revising for my "O" Levels and thought the countryside was so noisy with the cows mooing, the cockerels crowing and the sheep baaing! Of course I was more interested in boyfriends!

When I was in my twenties and thirties, I again enjoyed holidays with my own family. I have two children, Zoë and Nick and we took them on many camping holidays in Britain and also to France and Spain. We would do walks in Derbyshire, Yorkshire and the Lake District mostly. I would tempt them to the top of hills with Kendal mint cake! After the children left home, I started my own walking group as my day off from work was a Friday and I couldn't find a group that walked on Fridays. I advertised for ladies only as I thought it might be slightly risky to advertise for men! So the Lincolnshire Ladies Strolling Society was born. Everyone walked at a leisurely pace and we didn't go far, hence the name. I couldn't read maps at the time as I'd always been a follower rather than a leader so I used walking books and leaflets with local routes on. I then started to learn how to read maps but often went the wrong way. Sometimes we'd try to walk on a parish boundary! Often we'd need to wade through streams and climb fences when I'd gone wrong. So we changed the name to The Lincolnshire Ladies' Adventure Group as we were having so many unintentional adventures on our walks! And the name stuck. We always go away for two weekends a year usually to Derbyshire or Yorkshire. Some of us started to go away for a week's walking every year, often to Scotland.

It was two years ago in Melrose that my friends, Jacky, Linda and I saw an older lady, probably about my age, in her sixties, walking into our hotel. She was carrying a massive backpack including camping gear. Later that evening she sat near us in the restaurant. She was wolfing down great plate loads of food. Eventually we asked her where she was going. Her answer astounded me. She was walking from Land's End to John O' Groats! She'd been mostly camping but was exhausted and was taking a day off to rest and recover in this hotel. This encounter, though brief, was one of the motivations for me deciding to do this walk myself. Over the months that followed I kept thinking about her and what an amazing thing she was doing, walking on her own from Land's End to John O'Groats! Could I do it? It kept eating away at me, that memory and the thought that life was for living now. Being well again, I should do the walk to celebrate my health.

So I decided I would do it. It took me six months of happy planning. I borrowed and bought maps, forty seven in all! I spent hours poring over them and reading books about people who'd already done the walk, known as LeJog (Land's End to John O'Groats). There is no definitive route but Andrew McCloy's book, "From Land's End to John O'Groats", is very useful. He writes in detail about three possible routes, the Central route, West and East routes. I decided on the Central route to start with up to Horton in Ribblesdale then veer northwest to pick up the Western route to Fort William. After that I would go northeast to Inverness and finally finish by going up the east coast to John O'Groats. I loved the planning and organising. There was a little bubble of excitement inside me all the time. I wanted to try to join up long distance paths where possible and only walk on minor roads where necessary. I didn't want to walk on any major roads at all. I couldn't wait to get going! Different friends and family would join me from time to time bringing me maps and different items of clothing and take back maps I'd finished with and unnecessary items that I no longer needed. It would take three and a half months to walk and about half of that I'd be walking on my own. I was looking forward to being on my own as I love to take photos and like studying the wild flowers without feeling that companions may be impatient to move on.

I decided I would do it for Charity so I chose the local fund (for North East Lincolnshire) called "Drive for Grimsby" which raises money to help disadvantaged youngsters take part in the Duke of Edinburgh's Award Scheme. It's a marvellous organisation that gives young people more confidence and develops their skills. It fosters a love of the British countryside and a sense of adventure by taking them on walking and camping expeditions in Lincolnshire, Derbyshire and Yorkshire. They provide minibuses to take them out to the hills and provide tents, boots and waterproofs for those who can't afford them.

Ian and I started out on Easter Sunday 2017 for Land's End. He'd wanted to do all of it with me as he'd been doing contract work which was flexible but then he got a full time job so was only able to join me from time to time. We had a long journey by train from Grimsby, then by plane from Leeds Bradford Airport to Newquay which only took an hour, followed by three hours on buses, trains, a taxi and walking to get to Land's End. We got to the Land's End sign for the obligatory photo at 7pm. There were not too many people there. The sea and rocky promontory looked beautiful in the evening light.

My rucksack weighed 35lbs! I'd decided that despite advice to leave some stuff out, I couldn't possibly manage without its total contents. However by the time we'd walked the half mile or so to our B & B, I knew it was too heavy. I couldn't even lift it. Ian had to put it on me! The thick book that I'd saved to read all the way to John O'Groats was the first thing to go. It was left at the B & B for some lucky person to find. We'd booked a meal at a nearby pub but by the time we'd finished at Land's End it was too late to get a meal. Fortunately, the B & B was like a self-catering flat and there was food for breakfast in the fridge so we ate some of that for our evening meal.

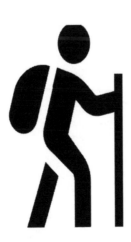

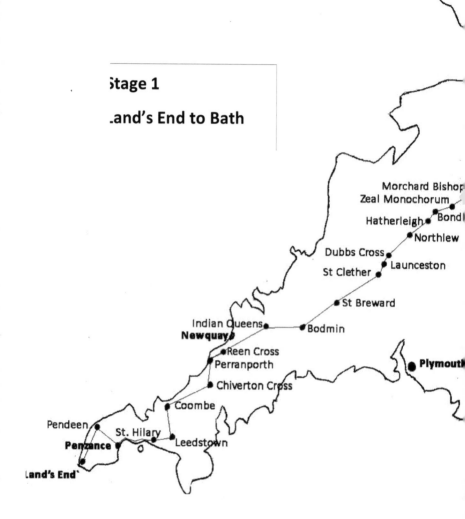

Stage 1

Land's End to Bath

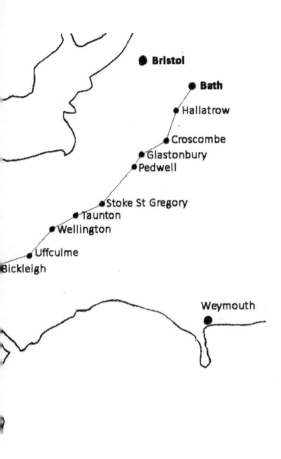

Bristol

Bath

Hallatrow

Croscombe

Glastonbury

Pedwell

Stoke St Gregory

Taunton

Wellington

Uffculme

Bickleigh

Weymouth

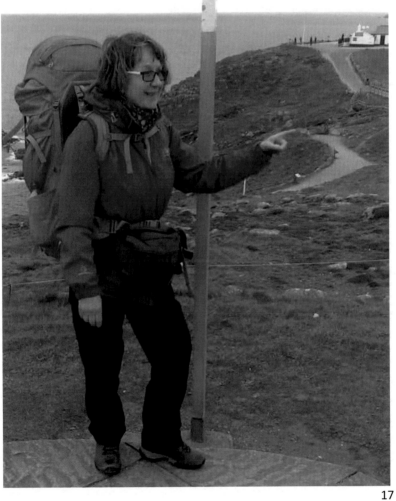

Stage 1   Land's End to Bath   16/4 – 11/5

		Ordinance Survey Map
Land's End to Pendeen	10 miles	Landranger 203
Pendeen to St. Hilary	15 miles	LR 203
St Hilary to Leedstown	8 miles	LR 203
Leedstown to Coombe	8 miles	LR 203
Coombe to Chiverton Cross	9 miles	LR 203
Chiverton Cross to Reen Cross Farm	6 miles	LR 204, 200 OS Explorer 106
Reen Cross Farm to Pengorse Farm	14 ½ miles	LR 200
Pengorse Farm to Bodmin	14 miles	LR 200
Bodmin to St Breward	10 ½ miles	LR 200
St Breward to St Clether	10 ½ miles	LR 200
St Clether to Launceston	10 miles	LR 201
Launceston to Dubbs Cross	11 miles	LR 190, 191
Dubbs Cross to Northlew	10 miles	LR 191
Northlew to Bondleigh	13 miles	Ex.113
Bondleigh to Morchard Bishop	12 miles	Ex. 113
Morchard Bishop to Bickleigh	14 miles	Ex.114
Bickleigh to Uffculme	14 miles	Ex.114
Uffculme to Wellington	11 miles	Ex.114
Wellington to Taunton	9 miles	Ex. 128
Taunton	Day off	
Taunton to Stoke St Gregory	11 miles	Ex.128
Stoke St Gregory to Pedwell	13 miles	Ex. 128, 140 & 141
Pedwell to Glastonbury	7 miles	Ex. 141
Glastonbury to Croscombe	8 ½ miles	Ex. 141
Croscombe to Hallatrow	13 miles	Ex.141
Hallatrow to Bath	16 miles	Ex. 142, 155
Bath	2 days off	
Total	**282 miles**	**25 walking days.**

Average 11.1 miles per day. Days off: 3

Easter Sunday April 16th

Land's End to Pendeen **Cornwall**   *10 miles*

It was a sunny morning as Ian and I set off from the B & B on my first day of the longest walk I've ever done. However I knew that the trick was to only think of one day at a time, never the whole tremendous journey that lay ahead.

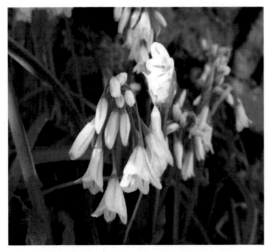

Wild garlic or Three-cornered leek

The roadside verges were so pretty, full of white flowers that I thought were white bluebells. The locals called it wild garlic. The only wild garlic I know is ramsons which grows mainly in woods. I've never seen this flower before. The banks were covered in bluebells, delicate white stitchwort and primroses. There was also golden gorse giving out its wonderful coconut aroma.

Despite the feast for my eyes and nose, the pain of carrying my massive rucksack marred the day. It was almost thirty five pounds despite leaving the big book at the B & B. Ian had to lift it onto me as I couldn't lift it! After several excruciating miles, Ian took five pounds off me into his rucksack. It was so much better but still not easy. My feet were singing and my right foot was hurting. But no blisters yet.

19

We took a more direct route than planned, by the coast to see Sennen Cove then along pretty lanes and fields. We had printed off a new route from the internet which goes through central Cornwall and Devon and visits all the interesting historical parts of the countryside. We decided not to do it as we could see that it also went up every hill too! We met two lovely donkeys that I would have liked to take with me to carry my pack and to ride! But they wouldn't come. We went through St Just and had a welcome cup of tea at the pub. Now we're in a lovely pub at Pendeen. And best of all….there's a bath! Perfect!

Monday April 17th

Pendeen to St Hilary   **Cornwall**   *15 miles*

We decided to send the two huge rucksacks ahead by taxi - £25, worth every penny! So today we travelled light and happy. Over the moors we saw Quoits. These are large stone constructions like huge tables supported by stone legs. Some were built about 5000 years ago and though some may have been used for burials, their primary use was probably for religious ceremonies. We saw Chun Castle, an ancient site which had a double stone wall surrounding a hill. We saw the many chimneys of the old tin mines which once made Cornwall rich, at least for the owners of the mines! It brought back memories of my favourite TV programme, Poldark.

We walked under archways of white blackthorn blossom and golden gorse through lanes and fields and over moors. Again there were lots of beautiful wild flowers and the weather continued to be fine. It was very hilly. I didn't know that Cornwall was so hilly. We walked to Penzance where Ian bought a long-sleeved T shirt as he got sunburnt yesterday. Found a café for tea and cake! We then walked along the coast path past stunning St Michael's Mount. My right foot was aching more and more. We had to walk along a road with no footpath for about a mile but reached the pub in a village near

20

our B & B and had a lovely meal – duck salad with figs, blue cheese and walnuts. Delicious! Our B & B is the Old Vicarage at St Hilary and it's lovely.

Tuesday April 18th

St Hilary to Leedstown **Cornwall** *8 miles*

Another sunny day. We walked along some lovely lanes with wild flowers of bluebells, primroses, stitchwort, garlic mustard and red campion. We faced our first challenge too. We were following a signed route across a field that suddenly had an electric fence going across the middle of it with no obvious way of getting round it. There was a clearly marked signpost the other side of the field. We decided to shimmy under the fence on our stomachs, commando style. The large rucksacks on our backs didn't help. (We should have taken them off really.) We were watched by a herd of amazed cows! When we reached the stone stile at the other side of the field I had to struggle over it as the downward route involved a leap of faith to avoid part of a broken ladder which had a dagger of metal sticking out. The pursuing bullocks that suddenly appeared behind me encouraged me greatly!

We enjoyed a lengthy lunch break at the side of the road, sunbathing. I changed into my shorts for the first time.

We're camping at Callose Campsite, our first night of camping. It's a lovely place. A friendly couple from Beverley gave us a cup of tea 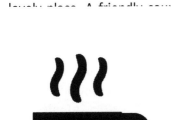 and invited us into their caravan. We walked to the pub and enjoyed a nice meal. As it's still lovely weather camping doesn't seem too bad at the moment.

Wednesday April 19th

Leedstown to Coombe campsite   **Cornwall**   *8 miles*

A night of hell! It was too cold and I kept slipping off the rolled out spongy mat that goes under the sleeping bag. The good thing was I didn't get up for the toilet for twelve hours! However, I hardly slept.

Today's fine again. We walked along a few roads and some lovely lanes. New flowers today were lousewort, a small purple flower, and comfrey (cream and red). I looked carefully at the difference between ramsons, which has a larger leaf and spiky starry flowers spread in a circle and the other wild garlic which smells more of spring onion and has a narrower leaf and several bell flowers drooping down. It is much more common than ramsons round here.

The highlight of today was going to a Horticultural College thinking there was a café there. However it's not really open to the public. There was only a shop to buy a drink and some bars to eat. This was opened especially for us. We were directed to a picnic bench in the middle of the lawn. We were enjoying our drink when two Rhode Island Red chickens appeared and showed a great interest in us, obviously not for our scintillating conversation but for our food. Despite my telling him not to, Ian, (a push over), gave them a bit of his biscuit bar. Then, as I was looking at Ian, the other chicken jumped up on the table and pecked the whole bar out of my hand and proceeded to eat it in front of me on the table! The cheek! It was very funny but disappointing as I'd only had one bite out of it and now the shop was closed.

Originally we were going to wild camp but as there are so many campsites in Cornwall and that I hate camping anyway, we decided to go to campsites. We found a campsite, Calloose. It is quite basic but adequate. Ian and I have swapped sleeping bags and mat as I found the bag too cold and the mat too slippery. I kept falling off it.

My feet felt better today. I put talc on them and wore one pair of thin socks and loosened the laces near the toes. My shoulders and back hurt though as the rucksack is still too heavy. I need to lighten it when possible.

Thursday April 20th

Magor Farm, Coombe to Chiverton Cross   **Cornwall**   *9 miles*

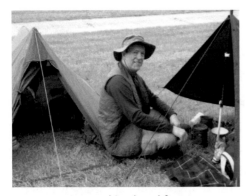

Ian cooking breakfast

The night was slightly better in the tent in the other sleeping bag. I still needed to wear two thermal vests, thermal long johns and a fleece jumper! I slept OK till midnight then the next four hours were not so good. There was the sound of a babbling brook next to us which was not conducive to trying not to go to the toilet. However, I managed to get through the night till 6am. Then I couldn't open the zip of the tent! And I still kept slipping off the mat. I hate camping so much! I only do it as it's cheap. I quite like eating the porridge that Ian makes in the morning and sitting in the sun eating it. What extra hell it will be if we get bad weather!

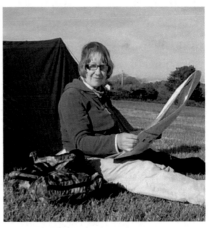

I'm studying the map

Today was another sunny day. We had a lovely walk through woodlands full of flowers. We found a Visitor Centre Café for coffee and cake. Marvellous! Then more lanes and some road walking but it was mostly quiet roads. My feet felt OK today but on arrival at The Chiverton Arms I discovered a blister on a toe.

The pub is wonderful. We had lovely food for our evening meal. I had fish pie with delicious vegetables followed by waffles with honey ice cream.

Friday April 21st

Chiverton Cross to Reen Cross Farm **Cornwall** *6 miles*

Lovely walking again in fine sunny weather through flower bedecked paths and lanes with little streams by the roadsides. We walked on a few quiet roads too. We went via Perranporth and at last had a Cornish cream tea! I'm going to try to eat the local delicacy of each county I go through if possible. The scone was very light with proper Cornish clotted cream and lovely strawberry jam.

Then we sat by the beach but there was a very cool wind which started to chill us as we sat there too long really. Actually it was very touristy but it was an attractive beach full of rocky outcrops. I had a few bites of Ian's Cornish pasty so that's two local delicacies in one day!

We then went to the Reen Cross Farm campsite which we found by ringing from the pub last night. It's not really open yet so no one's here except the owner, a nice young man called Craig who wants me to let him know when I get to John O'Groats. The toilets are spotless as it's brand new.

Saturday April 22nd

Reen Cross Farm to Pengorse Farm   **Cornwall**   *14 ½ miles*

It was a difficult day today due to a lot of road walking in the morning on busy roads. Sometimes we go on roads if we want to cover a good distance on the most direct route. The best bit of the walk was finding a pub at Mitchell where I had a lovely cauliflower and blue cheese soup for lunch. We only went down one beautiful flowery lane today. We saw an early purple orchid. We went in a lovely church at St Edinor which had the wild garlic flowers and bluebells in the churchyard. Today we saw ramsons and the Cornish wild garlic flowers growing close together.

We went to a nice Chinese restaurant at Indian Queens village a mile before the campsite, "Gnome World Caravan Site". My feet were really aching today especially the little toe that has the blister. I wrapped sheep's wool round my toes. We've booked a taxi tomorrow to take the rucksacks to Bodmin.

Sunday April 23rd

Pengorse Farm to Bodmin   **Cornwall**   *14 miles*

Another warm, sunny day. The taxi took the bags (£19) to Bodmin so it should have been a lovely day but my blistered toe gave me a lot of pain so I was hobbling most of the day.

We visited an Iron Age fort, Castle-An-Dinas, which was impressive and had superb views of Cornwall.

The ramsons flower seems to have taken over from the wild garlic one now. We saw a few wood anemones. The quiet roads were lovely. The approach to Bodmin was divine with the banks on the roadside absolutely covered with bluebells and ramsons as well as primroses, stitchwort and red campion. We heard a cuckoo as we

25

walked through a "Down". This was a Nature Reserve which had rough grass and gorse. We also heard willow warblers, chiff chaff, robins, skylarks and tits.

The pub where we're staying in Bodmin is very noisy. It's "Olde Worlde" in a nice way. We went to Wetherspoons for a good meal and a glass of wine.

Monday April 24th

Bodmin to St Breward **Cornwall** *10½ miles plus 1 mile for tomorrow's walk.*

The Camel Trail

Ian left to go home on the train. My friend Dawn, from my walking group, came to the White Hart Inn where we were staying and brought me a postcard to send to my grandsons, Kyriacos and Alexander, for their map of Great Britain that I had given them before I left to keep a track of where I am. Kyriacos is six and Alexander four. I'm planning to send them postcards regularly and

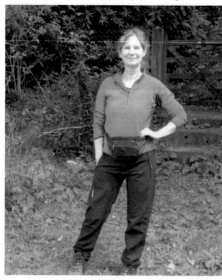

Dawn

my daughter, Zoë, will put a star on the route I have drawn on the map to show where I am. Then Dawn and I drove to Dunmere to start at where I'd got to yesterday. It was a beautiful, easy walk (for a change), along the Camel Trail by a river. However the blister on my toe killed me. I was hobbling. We went to a lovely café and had a Cornish cream tea. We saw a black cap singing really

26

close to us. It was so nice to be chatting to Dawn.

It's always good to walk with Dawn as she has a great knowledge of nature, especially birds and insects. There was a bit of minor road walking to St Breward then I did an extra mile of tomorrow's walk over attractive fields.

We climbed two Cornish stone stiles. These are very different to any stiles I've seen before. They consist of a series of large stones separated by gaps which can be up to two feet deep. They usually rise up and down like steps. I found them quite scary at first as there's nothing to hold onto at the side and with a heavy pack on, you can overbalance. We also saw the wild garlic flowers again that we

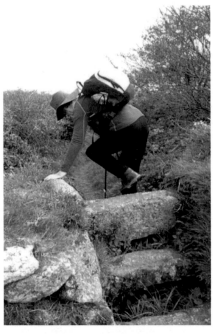

I'm struggling over a Cornish stile.

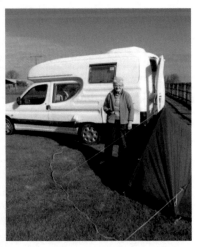

thought had been taken over by the ramsons. Dawn drove us then to Newquay where I stayed with her and her family in a large mobile home. It was lovely. I had my own tiny bedroom! I was able to soak my aching feet for ages in hot water. I'm happy!

Patsy with her camper van and tent

Tuesday April 25th

St Breward to St Clether **Cornwall** *10 ½ miles (Less 1 mile which I did yesterday)*

Dawn drove us to St Brewards where we finished yesterday. The weather has changed today. It's bitterly cold with snow and hail! Today's walk started with a very high difficult stile that I couldn't manage. I'd thrown my poles over. Dawn was ahead so couldn't help. I had to go round the field until I found a gate which I climbed and went back down a lane to retrieve my poles. Then I met up with Dawn and we crossed fields with ponies and horses wandering onto the quiet roads. They didn't bother us. I'm afraid of most animals. I've got more confidence if I'm with someone. There were not so many flowers today.

Davidson Woods and disused airfield was very open, cold and bleak. We met Patsy, my older sister, just before St Clether. Patsy is coming to join me for a week in her camper van. Patsy adores cats. She always takes her cat with her on holidays but Jessica is a new cat, not used to going in camper vans and unfortunately, she has not taken to Patsy.

Patsy told me that on arrival in Wells, (about three hours' drive from here), she tried to get the halter on Jessica with her contact details on but she struggled so much that in the end Patsy gave up. Jessica escaped and ran away! However Patsy gave the farmer's wife food to leave out for her and in a week's time Patsy will go back to look for her.

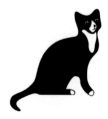

Wednesday April 26th

St Clether to Launceston   **Cornwall**   *10 miles*

It was a chilly start to the day as Patsy joined me for a mile along some lanes. Then we had a difficult gate to climb. It was leaning forward a bit which always makes it tricky. However, we both managed it. Patsy does very well as she is nearly 80! However she is a seasoned walker, having walked round the entire coast of Britain when she was 60 and in more recent years has walked the length and breadth of France! So I'm continuing a family tradition of walkers! Then we came to a farm where a sheep dog was barking at us and accompanied us out of the farmyard. I used my loving dog voice that my friend, Jacky, has tutored me in. It seemed to work. Then we walked through a cow field, around a bog and climbed another gate. At this point, Patsy went back to the camper van and met me at the end of the walk.

A lovely part of the walk came then, along very quiet roads with beautiful trees and woods at the side of the roads. I went into the wood and sat on a log for a drink and a biscuit. The sun came out though it was still chilly. I was happy.

At Egloskerry I was looking forward to walking along the river on a disused railway line but I couldn't access it. I went to a house next to where I thought the access point was but was told it was now privately owned. Also I had to walk on a "B" road which was quite unpleasant with traffic for nearly five miles. However there were panoramic views.

Launceston came into view with a castle and a church on top of a hill. My feet were aching. I reached the town and asked about finding a café that served cream teas. I was told they were at the top of the hill. Typical! So I didn't get one.

I met Patsy in the camper van and after some shopping at the Co-op we went to the campsite. Patsy cooked me a stir-fry and I enjoyed wine and chocolate! Patsy is in her tiny tent as she loves camping and I sleep in the camper van which is better than being in a tent but still not good. The bench seat I sleep on is too narrow and my sleeping bag is made of nylon and the blankets keep slipping off it. And the camper van is the smallest they make so it's a challenge when we both are in it. One person has to lie on the bench so the other person can move around. But I'm grateful for the help Patsy is giving me. She is a very kind sister.

Thursday April 27th

Launceston to Dubbs Cross **Devon** *11 miles*

The Two Castles Trail

This was a cool day and a day of getting lost both walking and driving! First of all Patsy and I couldn't find the way to walk out of Launceston. Villages and towns are often quite tricky to negotiate on foot. After going round and round, we eventually found the way and Patsy went back to the camper van to join me at the end of the day's walk.

I crossed the wide River Tamar and entered Devon. I was following the path of the Two Castles Trail but because I forgot my binoculars I couldn't see where the exit of the path was in the huge field. On checking my GPS I discovered I was too far west. So I went east and entered a wood which I just about encircled. There was no way out that I could find. There was a river to one side and fences all round so it was very difficult to go in the right direction according to my compass. Eventually I climbed two fences and went through a hole in a fence. Then I climbed a hill and exited to the correct road through a gap in the hedge which was covered with thick branches. I threw my rucksack down to the road which was about three yards down as it was one of the many Devon roads with steep banks. After that I managed to squeeze past the thorns and branches, jumped off a rock and landed on the road! Phew!

Finally I had to walk along a long minor road to the pub at St Giles on the Heath. There was a very pleasant lady publican there who used to live in Lincoln. Despite it being 3pm closing time, she gave me a coffee and two chocolates and two of the male customers gave me £15 between them for my charity when they found out what I was doing. I walked four more miles to reduce tomorrow's walk length. New flowers today were common vetch and cuckoo flower.

Patsy met me and we headed on a long route to a new campsite near Brideswell, for me a somewhat overstimulating drive. The hilly, winding and narrow roads of Devon are difficult to drive on at the best of times. In a camper van where the driver, blessed by shortness and a seat that will not move forward, is ergonomically challenged to reach the pedals the excitement is intensified. As we approached the top of a hill in Launceston, the van stalled and slipped back a bit – to the consternation of myself, Patsy and following drivers. Frankly I was terrified. I gently encouraged Patsy with words that were probably as much for myself as her. I had to believe that I would survive, after all I still had 1100 miles to go.

The antithesis of Jeremy Clarkson, being chauffeured by Patsy is a unique and special experience for a privileged few; a must for any adrenaline junkies looking for extreme alternatives to extreme activities. Choosing to remain within the confines of the law, Patsy has put her days of driving like a dragster racer behind her, preferring the calmness of a very sedate Sunday outing and leading what sounds like a flock of geese as drivers following her honk encouragingly. Sometimes the geese may annoy Patsy who will exclaim at them in a language I do not understand, "merde!" and other fancy words.

Friday April 28th

Dubbs cross to Northlew **Devon** *10 miles*

I walked fast on minor roads today as my blister wasn't causing me any pain. Then I was on a footpath which led through a farm where a large dog started barking at me and came up to me. I was very nervous but did the "loving" voice that Jacky taught me and it stopped barking but escorted me all the way to the edge of the farm property. I breathed a sigh of relief when I got through the gate. However, when I glanced back, there it was, still with me. It must have gone round the side somehow. It decided it would join me. For the next two miles it accompanied me through fields and woods. I ignored it, hoping it would go back. Eventually I came to a gate. I went through it quickly but soon found the dog with me again. It must have found a gap to get through. At the next gate, there were definitely no gaps. I rushed through but I think it must have jumped over! It was still with me! After another mile, we reached a gate and on the other side I saw there were lambs. I knew how important it was not to let the dog near the lambs. Dogs can be shot for worrying sheep. So I decided to climb this one to make sure the dog didn't follow. It peered at me soulfully through the bars of the gate. I shouted at it to go home. Eventually it did. What a relief!

As if that wasn't enough, a bit later I entered another farm yard and two black Labradors rushed up to me, barking. Luckily a man in a barn nearby shouted to them and they calmed down. I wish I wasn't so frightened of dogs. I have to be brave.

I walked through some lovely woodlands today and by a lake. The new flower that I saw today was bugle. I also saw the wild Cornish garlic flower again but not in abundance. At last, after many more hilly, narrow, winding roads, I reached Northlew. It's a very pretty village with thatched roof cottages and a village cross. There's a lovely church dedicated to Thomas of Canterbury. When Patsy arrived, we had a coffee in the pub and a man gave me a donation of £20. People are so kind.

The campsite at Winkleigh is very basic. There's no Wi-Fi and no hook up and the toilet and shower are in a barn and look awful. The tap for the shower is yards away on an outside wall. The toilet has no light. So we didn't go in and just used the toilet in the camper van and cleaned our teeth in a mug. There's no other campers here, just some alpacas in a field over the fence on the other side to where we are camping. The ground is quite uneven with long grass. We were going to stay two nights here but we've told the man in charge we only want one night. Patsy has just come into the camper van to spend the night in here with me. She was settling down to sleep when she heard heavy breathing outside the tent!

Saturday April 29th

Northlew to Bondleigh **Devon** *13 miles*

Another morning search for the next campsite; another interesting drive. I had found out that Patsy was waiting for cataract treatment and this morning she drove with extra care so as not to miss the signs advertising flowers, eggs, potatoes, cafes and so on. With my fingers drawing blood from my palms, my desperate pleas for *me* to check the signs so that she could concentrate on driving went unheeded. Eventually we found a site – a field; no toilet, no shower, just a cold tap - life really doesn't get better than this, so I refused it believing myself undeserving.

Patsy took me to Northlew and a Mars ice-cream bar helped restore my shattered nerves – she's an angel in disguise. I started my walk at 12.30pm and Patsy continued the search for another campsite more suited to the undeserving and unappreciative of the simple pleasures in life.

The walk was lovely and I walked fast. It was all minor roads with great views of the countryside and Dartmoor in the distance. It was very hilly. At one point, a lady driver stopped her car to chat to me about where I was going and what I was doing. A car had to stop behind her while she chatted. He wasn't impatient at all. He just waited! Amazing!

I got to Hatherleigh after five miles and unfortunately found that the only café was shut. So I went in the George Pub. The barmaid was impressed when I told her what I was doing as she volunteers for the Scouts so appreciated the work of the Duke of Edinburgh's Award Scheme for young people that I'm raising money for. I enjoyed a coffee and a delicious plate of sweet potato chips.

At Monkokehampton I sat on a seat to rest opposite one of the many beautiful thatched cottages and a lady came out to offer me a cup of tea and a bar of chocolate! Her husband then came out and asked me if I was going to John O'Groats. I said "yes" but how did he know? He said that's where the walkers usually sat who were going to John O'Groats. Amazing!

Another five miles took me to Bondleigh. It was a delightful walk. I saw orchids and scurvygrass which, despite its name, is a very pretty white flower, as well as the usual flowers.

Patsy had found a good campsite and we celebrated with a bottle of Rioja.

Sunday April 30th

Bondleigh to Morchard Bishop   ***Devon***   *12 miles*

The Two Moors Way

This was the first rainy day since I started my walk. I've been very lucky with the weather. It rained steadily all morning. I arrived like a drowned rat at Zeal Monochorum pub. It was very posh but welcoming which I think is always a good sign of a quality place when they welcome you despite your appearance. I had a delicious tomato and basil soup with warm bread and coffee. I spent an hour there, writing my article for the Cleethorpes Chronicle (I send them an update of my progress every week) as there was free Wi-Fi.

The rain eased off in the afternoon. I went on the Two Moors Way footpath but went wrong so diverted to a road for a while. Three dogs rushed to me on a road by a farm but they were fine and didn't bark. Then I saw a lady with two children and two dogs on the footpath near some woods. One of the dogs took a dislike to me but luckily she put it on a lead.

Monday May 1st

Morchard Bishop to Bickleigh   ***Devon***   *14 miles*

It was a difficult day today. There were steep hills and at one point I was going along a footpath through some fields and woods when I came across a sign which read "To Scotland". Well, I thought, that's very helpful as that's where I'm going. However I checked the map and found it was actually going to Scotland Copse. Then I followed another footpath sign which ended at a river! There was no way I was going to cross it as it looked quite deep, so I had to make a long diversion round.

I came to two fields of bullocks. In the first field they looked at me and ran the other way! That made a pleasant change! In the second field which I found joined the previous one with a gap, the same bullocks ran towards me to have a closer look. I made the gate before they did! I had to shelter from a heavy shower in one church and lay down on a pew to recover from exhaustion in another church.

At the end of the day just before I was being met by Patsy in the camper van, I discovered my rucksack had been open at the back and I'd been dropping things along the road. Patsy arrived shortly after and we drove slowly back and soon found the things I'd dropped. We stopped at a wonderful location, a cafe next to the River Exe with a lovely bridge. We sat outside in the sun enjoying a well-deserved Devon cream tea.

Tuesday May 2nd

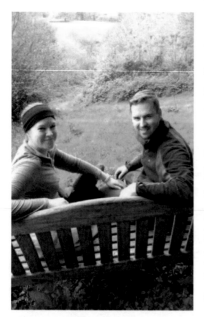

Kat and Nick

Bickleigh to Uffculme
Devon   *14 miles*

Today my son Nick and his wife Kat came to walk with me for two days. They are staying at a B & B a few miles away. It was great to see them and catch up with all their news. It was quite hard today, very hilly in the morning. I went wrong twice with the navigating. We had lunch on a seat with lovely views but discovered it was the wrong place and had to go back. We saw two lovely donkeys and two fox cubs playing.

We arrived at Cullompton and immediately saw a café and had a delicious Devon cream tea. The afternoon walk was much flatter and easier and on roads at first. Then we enjoyed a beautiful walk along the river Culme. Patsy met us and walked the last mile with us.

Wednesday May 3rd

Uffculme to Wellington **Devon** *11 miles*

Nick, Kat and I had a great walk along the River Culme to Culmstock. We found an interesting café for coffee and cake. The cloakroom was decorated with sheets of music on the walls, a violin, the inside pieces of a piano and groups of piano keys with their hammers! It was fascinating, especially to Nick and I who are musicians.

The next part of the walk was quite tough, climbing through deep, black, muddy paths in a forest. However the climb was worth it as we ended up on a grassy plateau with superb views. We walked by the Wellington Monument and under the M5 motorway. We met Patsy in Wellington.

Thursday May 4th

Wellington to Taunton **Somerset** *9 miles*

Patsy left today to continue her journey to see friends and to return to Wells to try to find her cat, Jessica. I tried to go on a footpath but lost confidence in my navigation so retraced my steps and took a back road option instead. I found a nice pub for lunch. There was no café in the first village but I bought an ice cream from the village shop. On telling the shopkeeper what I was doing, she gave me £2 for my charity. So kind!

After lunch, I had a scary experience going through a field of bullocks. At first I thought they were just friendly cows as they were all sitting down but they started to get up when they saw me and follow me. There were about forty of them and they followed me closely. I was very nervous as they are so big and can be unpredictable, although they are probably just bored and looking for a bit of fun to liven their day. A group of them started to stampede alongside me. I turned and shouted at them in my fiercest voice, waving my arms in the air. They seemed to have decided to do a pincer movement to block off my exit at the gate. There was no escape as next to me was an electric fence and a river. I kept up a fast walk as I knew you weren't supposed to run and I continued shouting at them. I just made it to the gate before they did! Phew!

After that I daren't go on my planned footpath route and went on minor roads to Taunton via another pub for a coffee to recover. I'm now staying at a comfortable B & B, Heathercroft, in Taunton. Heaven!

Friday May 5th

Taunton **Somerset** *Day off. 4 miles sauntering around.*

I'm playing a hand pan.

It was chilly today. I cleaned my boots. I walked into Taunton and found the canal where I'll walk tomorrow. I visited the museum and did part of the Town Trail.

I met a busker, Elliot, playing an interesting instrument. I watched him for a while then gave him a pound. We started chatting and he told me the instrument was a hand pan, related to the steel drum but you sit on the ground to play it with your hands. He let me have a go.

I didn't manage to earn any money for him but on telling him about my charity walk he gave me back the pound I'd given him! Then I chatted to a lap harp player. I was particularly interested as I have a lap harp at home on which I occasionally play some very simple arrangements of carols at Christmas. He was playing some very intricate and beautiful arrangements of Irish music. Ian arrived in the evening for the weekend. We risked fish and chips from a shop. It was nice but very expensive compared with Grimsby prices. And not as good as Grimsby fish and chips, naturally. It was great to see Ian especially as he's brought his guitar to play to me.

Saturday May 6th

Taunton to Stoke St Gregory   **Somerset**   *11 miles*

Ian drove to Stoke St Gregory and walked towards me. He met me halfway then walked back with me to Stoke St Gregory.

I walked through Taunton hoping to see Elliot, the busker, but he wasn't in his usual place, probably too early for him. I went to the canal that I had found on my Taunton recce yesterday and had a pleasant walk along the canal towpath. I was confused as to the right way near the motorway but orientated the map to the ground and got it right.

At the pub at Creech St Michael where I had a coffee, the man at the bar, the only customer apart from me, started chatting and on finding out what I was doing gave me £5. Then the barmaid, called Yana, after the singer of long ago, gave me £2.

I walked along a minor road through Ham and then away from the canal over fields where I met Ian for a picnic lunch. We're now in the Somerset Levels which is a great relief after all the hills. The canals and the long straight roads have beautiful white cow parsley and yellow rape flowers on the verges all the way along. It's so pretty! This is a willow growing area and we passed a shop selling willow baskets and other willow ornaments but unfortunately it had just closed.

On walking by the canal again where the long fields go right up to the water, we had an unpleasant experience. There were several fields where the bullocks ran up to us. We raised our arms which usually slows them down momentarily. However the worst was a group containing a bull with a ring in its nose! They ran towards us and despite knowing you shouldn't run we ran as fast as we could and reached the gate just before them. Usain Bolt would have been proud of us! It was so scary. I was glad Ian was with me. I've decided to try to walk on roads more.

We're staying at the Rose and Crown Pub at Stoke St Gregory. It's wonderful. There is a massive bath. Just what you need for an aching body. We ate a lovely meal and we had cider too!

Sunday May 7th

Stoke St Gregory to Pedwell   **Somerset**   *13 miles*

It's been a lovely warm day today with no cows or bullocks, although this morning when I was alone on a road, a farmer on a quad bike stopped me as he said cows were coming along the road. I retreated well back. But when they appeared round the bend there were just two docile cows!

Ian walked from Pedwell to meet me halfway at Westonzoyland, a lovely village with a church and a pub. We enjoyed easy walking along lanes and through villages. It was flat as we're still in the Somerset Levels. There was an interesting moment when I saw a horse and cart coming along the road with a family in it and two dogs, tied on with leads, trotting along beside them. They looked very happy, probably renting it for a few days holiday. Then we saw an enormous steam engine, black and gleaming, probably off to a show as it's a Sunday. We had a picnic in a sunny churchyard and a drink in the pub. There were lovely footpaths in the afternoon and no bullocks. We saw two small deer, possibly muntjacs. A blackcap sang to us from a tree and we also heard sedge warblers, a cuckoo, chiffchaffs, wrens and robins.

We walked through fields of buttercups and by canals and dykes bordered with yellow rape flowers.

The wild garlic flowers appeared again in a village before Pedwell and a local confirmed that they were the garlic flower and it grew around this area, but I've not seen anymore.

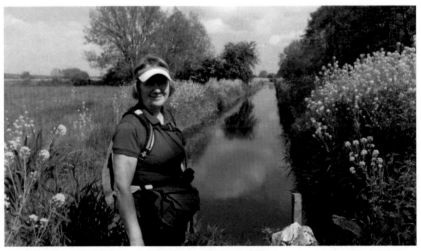

In the Somerset Levels

My little toe is in a poor state from the blister, red and swollen. The nail seems dead and may come off. I have two more blisters on two other toes too.

I've heard from Patsy. On arriving back at Wells she went to see the farmer's wife who'd been leaving out food for Jessica, Patsy's missing cat. She told Patsy that Jessica was probably in the barn. She was! However, as the cat doesn't like Patsy she wouldn't come to her and ran off. They eventually traced her to someone's greenhouse in a garden. All this had taken about three hours! The owner of the greenhouse said she would get Jessica. She went in to the greenhouse and within a few minutes she came out with a purring Jessica in her arms! Jessica was eventually put back in the camper van and taken back to York, protesting all the way! She'd had such a good time on her adventure!

Monday May 8th

Pedwell to Glastonbury   **Somerset**   *7 miles*

It was another great day today with sunny and warm weather. It helped a lot that Ian took my big bag to the B & B at Glastonbury for me on his way home. So I only carried my small rucksack today. I had an easy walk along little roads and some footpaths with no beasts. I walked through a Nature Reserve where I heard reed warblers. In one village that I went through, I played a lovely piano in the church as there was nobody in it. And I nearly joined in a Line Dancing class when I popped into the Village Hall to go to the toilet.

I arrived in Glastonbury at lunchtime in glorious sunshine after taking it slowly and stopping to rest twice in the sunshine. I could see the famous Tor, the hill with the tower of a ruined medieval church on top. There was no way I wanted to climb it. I've done enough hills in Devon and Cornwall and I thought I'd better save my strength for more to come!

I entered Glastonbury and went in the first café I came across. It was vegetarian and had a hippy look to it, as did the owner, dressed in a flowing dress. I had a delicious cake and an interesting apricot tea served in a samovar. I continued into the square in the town centre. Looking round I realised that all the shops were alternative, selling hippy, Indian clothes or mystical artefacts. There were aromatherapy and herbal boutiques too. A lot of people were wearing hippy clothes, even the old ones. I felt as if I'd been transported back to the 60's!

I had a guided tour of the ruined Abbey by a guide dressed as a monk. He was very good and it was interesting. The Abbey is reputed to be the final resting place of King Arthur and Queen Guinevere! Afterwards, I lay on the grass in the parkland sunbathing for ages. Then I went back to the first café and had a korma and flatbread for my tea. Delicious!

I found the way to my B & B, "The Moon in the Apple", (a typical Flower Power era name), which was in an old terrace cottage. My bedroom was lovely but my bathroom was basically a cupboard on the landing with a cold shower! The water went warm for a few seconds, enough to wet me, and then reverted to cold. Very annoying!

However, the next morning I had a delightful breakfast cooked in front of me by the owner, a beautiful young Flemish lady dressed in flowing trousers and embroidered top. The amazing kitchen was decorated with dried hops and flowers and the branches on the ceiling were hung with crystals. I had summer porridge which was oats soaked in orange juice over night with fresh strawberries and blueberries. My breakfast of eggs and tomatoes was cooked in front of me on the Aga. It was all so lovely that I forgave her the cold shower which she apologised for and said they were possibly washing up!

Tuesday May 9th

Glastonbury to Croscombe   **Somerset**   *8 ½ miles*

The first half of the walk today was lovely and easy on long, straight, flat roads with yellow rape flowers and clouds of white Queen Anne's lace flowers on either side. There were dykes each side too and fields with bullocks the other side of them so they couldn't get to me! I carried my heavy rucksack, now down to 28lbs as Ian and Patsy have taken some of the excess stuff away. And I was OK at first. Eventually though I had to stop every hour to rest and take my boots off. Then it became hilly. I missed a woodland path because I couldn't find out how to access it. I got very tired and despondent. Eventually I rang the B & B as I couldn't find it. I'd been given the wrong address, Old Road instead of Old Street Lane. However it was not too far away. Her house is amazing. It's a very big, old white cottage. My room is delightful. It is cosy and comfortable and decorated in an "olde worlde" but stylish way. Not at all like a hotel room would be. More like your own bedroom from long ago. There's also a magnificent wardrobe. I have my own bathroom and the run of the house! The lady sat with me when I arrived and gave me a cup of tea and chocolate biscuits while she chatted with me. Later I walked down the hill to the pub for my evening meal. Feeling very happy now.

Wednesday May 10th

Croscombe to Hallatrow   **Somerset**   *13 miles*

I had another very lovely and enjoyable day today in warm and sunny weather. The breakfast was unusual as it was a family breakfast with Kathy (the hostess) eating with me and the other guests, a French couple. Everyone chatted together and before I left, Kathy gave me £5 for my charity. The monster bag is being taken on by a taxi today (£15).

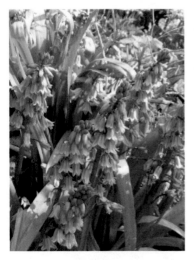

Bluebells

I'm now in the Mendip Hills so it was a hilly walk but not too steep, more like the Lincolnshire Wolds. There were some very quiet roads that I walked on and also some footpaths through a wooded area full of ramsons, (wild garlic). I walked through many beautiful buttercup fields. There were no beasts at all! The flowers that I'm seeing now are bush vetch, bluebells, stitchwort, red campion, bugle, cowslips and yellow archangel.

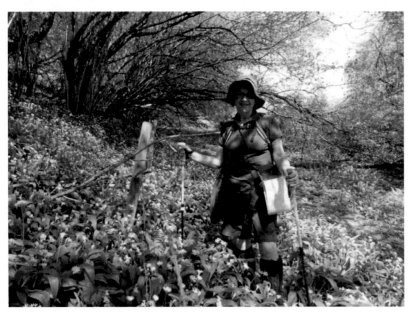

Walking through ransoms, wild garlic.

At 11am, I found a café in a garden centre for coffee and cake and at 12pm, a pub for cider and crisps! It doesn't usually happen like that. Later, I lay in a buttercup field in the sun watching a fox and her two cubs.

I arrived at the Station Inn at Hallatrow at 5pm and my rucksack was delivered shortly afterwards. My evening meal was spent in an old railway carriage in the pub garden. It was superb, like the inside of the Orient Express. There was piped classical piano music playing and wonderful food.

Thursday May 11th

Hallatrow to Bath   **Somerset**   *16 miles*

Avril and Mike arrived first thing in the morning after my non breakfast. The Pub, despite having wonderful evening meal arrangements, did not do breakfast. I made do with a coffee and biscuits from my room. Avril is my oldest friend. We met when we were eleven years old at school. Avril's husband Mike walked with us for a couple of miles.

We went on the Limestone Link path but there were difficulties in finding the paths. There were some stunning views. At one point, we got lost in someone's garden due to lack of signs. We went on a woodland trail ending in a steep, precipitous, gravelly slope and we suddenly recalled that at the start there'd been a sign telling people to avoid it so we did, (after Avril had started to go down it!)

We took an alternative route. We went through a field of bullocks that were quite calm and ignored us! We eventually decided it would be quicker to go on minor roads. It was very hilly.

My feet were killing me the last couple of hours. At about 5pm, we found a pub open for a welcome cup of tea.

In Bath, we unfortunately chose the wrong road to go down to find the Youth Hostel. It was a long road and we were very tired. We had to return uphill and eventually found the right road and the Youth Hostel. It's a grand old mansion set in large grounds. Mike came to collect Avril and they left me. I had a shower and a poor meal. There are no good meals on offer in Youth Hostels nowadays. My private room is like a prison cell. But the bathroom is nice.

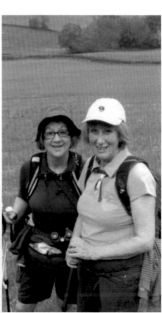

I'm with Avril

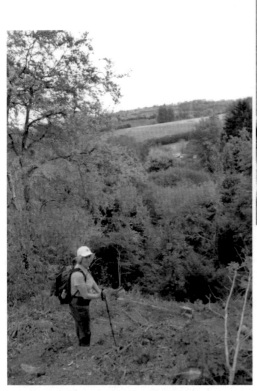

Avril starts the precipitous descent

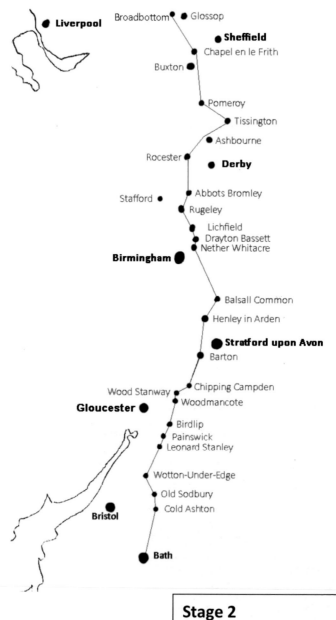

Stage 2

Bath to Broadbottom

Stage 2   **Bath to Broadbottom**   **12/5 – 8/6**

		Ordinance Survey Map
Bath to Cold Ashton	10 miles	Explorer 155
Cold Ashton to Old Sodbury	8 miles	Ex. 155
Old Sodbury to Wotton-under-Edge	10 miles	Ex.167
Wotton-under-Edge to Leonard Stanley	13 miles	Ex. 168 and 167
Leonard Stanley to Painswick	10 miles	Ex. 179
Painswick to Birdlip	8 miles	Ex. 179
Birdlip to Woodmancote	12 miles	Ex. 179
Woodmancote to Wood Stanway	8 miles	Ex. 179 & OL 45
Wood Stanway to Chipping Campden	11 miles	Ex. OL 45
Chipping Campden	Day off	
Chipping Campden to Barton	13 miles	Ex. OL 45 & Ex. 205
Barton to Henley-in-Arden	15 miles	Ex. OL 45 & Ex.220
Henley-in-Arden to Balsall Common	10 ½ miles	Ex. 220 & Ex. 221
Balsall Common to Nether Whitacre	15 miles	Ex. 221
Nether Whitacre to Drayton Bassett	8 miles	Ex. 221 and Ex. 220
Drayton Bassett to Lichfield	10 miles	Ex. 232 & Ex. 244
Lichfield to Castle Ring	10 miles	Ex. 244
Castle Ring to Abbots Bromley	13 miles	Ex. 259
Abbots Bromley to Rocester	16 ½ miles	Ex. 244 & Ex. 259
Rocester to Tissington	12 miles	Ex. 259
Tissington to Pomeroy	13 miles	Ex. 259 & Ex. OL24
Pomeroy to near Chapel-en-le-Frith	16 miles	Ex. OL24 & OL1
Near Chapel-en-le-Frith to Broadbottom	13 miles	Ex. OL1
Total	**255 miles**	**23 walking days**

Average 11.6 miles per day. Days off: 1

Friday May 12th   2 days off.

Bath.   Acton Turville.

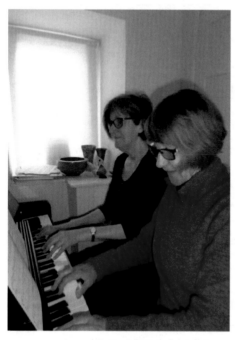

Chris and I played duets

My old friend Chris came to fetch me from the Youth Hostel at Bath for two days rest and recuperation at her house in the Cotswold village of Acton Turville. It was such a joy to see her and her husband Laurie and also her daughter Hannah and son Theo who popped in for a catch up. Theo played some jazz on the piano which was quite inspiring. It was great to see Chris's son John, who came all the way from Wales.

Chris and I played duets on the piano which was wonderful after so long on the road without live music.   We laughed at Hannah's reminiscence of her and my daughter Zoë's expedition to the Lake District when they were seventeen. Zoë had organised it and had drawn a line across the map showing the route they would walk. They noticed it crossed one of the lakes, Ullswater. So when they went, they carried a small inflatable boat and an oar each! Hannah was nervous about crossing the deep lake and had to be bribed with Opal fruits! They were famous during that holiday as people would hear about it or actually saw them crossing the lake, Hannah in the boat with the rucksacks and Zoë swimming behind. "There they are!" people would point and call out to each other. So you can see that this walking madness is a family trait!

Saturday May 13th

Acton Turville   Bath

Chris took me back to the Youth Hostel at Bath where I met Linda and Jacky who were going to walk the Cotswold Way with me, all one hundred and two miles of it. It was so lovely to see them and Jacky lent me her spare boots, size six, one size bigger than I normally take. It was like heaven putting them on! They felt like slippers. No rubbing on my blistered toes and room to wiggle and spread. We walked down the hill into the centre and saw the Royal Crescent and other iconic features. We had a delicious pie in a pub and walked back up the hill to the Youth Hostel.

Sunday May 14th

Bath to Cold Ashton (Cornflake Cottage, Pennsylvania)

Somerset and South Gloucestershire   12 miles

The Cotswold Way

Linda, Jacky and I set off on a sunny day from the Abbey in Bath to do the Cotswold Way. It took over two hours to reach the countryside. We had a coffee at a Golf place in Bath. We went through some fields of bullocks that ignored us completely. That made a change! The paths were very well marked and well kept.

On reaching a Garden Centre we met the crabby owner who was much too busy to get us a cup of tea so we helped ourselves. However, she was a wild flower expert. I quickly got out my camera and showed her the photo of the Cornish wild garlic flower. Despite her being very busy, she managed to reluctantly tell us that it was called the three-cornered leek. It was an introduction from Europe in the mid 1800's that has taken over in the South West. I was thrilled that at last I'd found out what it was. All parts of the plant are edible and it's known as an invasive plant. Well I think it's beautiful. Other flowers we saw today were wild mignonette (possibly), sweet woodruff and bird's-foot-trefoil.

My feet felt very comfortable in Jacky's boots but after a rain shower I discovered they're not waterproof. Tomorrow I'll wear my waterproof socks.

On approaching Cold Ashton Jacky slipped and fell on a gravelly path. She was shocked and bruised but was able to carry on.

Diane, the very nice B & B owner, gave me £30 for my charity! She took us to a lovely pub for a meal where you could order half portions. Such a good idea! Then you've got room for a pudding. I had pear and stilton salad followed by sticky toffee pudding with a butterscotch sauce and ice cream. It was very good.

I have a lovely double room to myself with a lace canopy. We're taking it in turns to have the best room if we're not together in one room.

Monday May 15th

Cold Ashton to Old Sodbury   **Gloucestershire**   *8 miles*

It was a cool, rainy day today but the rain was not heavy. It was a lovely walk with attractive scenery and not many hills for a change.

We found a café for coffee and cake at Dyrham Park but decided not to look round the house and garden as we didn't want to pay the fee. The woods were white with ransoms and the aroma of the wild garlic filled the air. At lunchtime we went in a church and I had a little play on the organ.

We're staying at The Dog Inn at Old Sodbury in a family room. The evening meal was good. I had cauliflower cheese and apple tart. The local delicacy for this county is Double Gloucester cheese which I savoured.

Tuesday May 16th

Old Sodbury to Wotton-under-Edge **Gloucestershire** *10 miles*

It rained on and off all day today. I had another comfortable day in Jacky's boots and we are having our bags carried every day by a baggage carrier so that's another great relief.

On our route we went through some pleasant woodland areas full of ramsons flowers and also passed a lovely old school. You have to

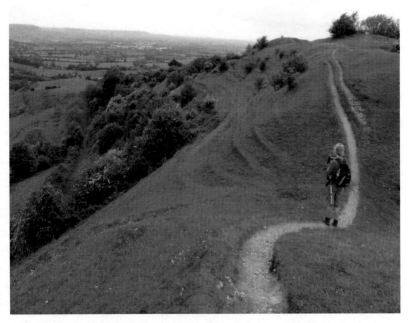

Jacky looks at terracing on the side of the hill.

be rich to live round here I think. We went by a perfect old house with its own lake and bridge which we crossed. There were swans on the lake.

The Cotswold Way goes through some historic areas with iron-age hill forts and Neolithic long barrows. There are monuments commemorating battles too. We passed some of them and there would have been some good views but it was too misty today.

The fields that we walked through had docile horses and cattle. I think they daren't misbehave in such a posh area!

We're staying in a lovely pub, The Swan, in a triple room. We like to stay together if possible. We're all good sleepers usually and none of us snore so it's good fun being together, as well as being cheaper. Wotton-under-Edge is quite a big village and it's attractive.

Wednesday May 17th

Wotton- under- Edge to Leonard Stanley **Gloucestershire**   *13 miles*

There was steady rain all day today. It was the worst day weather wise that I've had since Land's End. We went through some lovely woods though there were some big hills to climb. We saw two new flowers in the woods. One was a metre high with tiny pale creamy yellow bell shaped delicate flowers all down the stem. I don't know what it is. The other was large cuckoo pint. It has no spots on the leaves and it only grows in the south.

We passed by barrows and forts as usual and monuments. It got quite cold with all the rain. I put my poncho on too late as I was already quite wet. The turquoise anorak that I was wearing I can safely say is not waterproof. Despite having the wrists tightly fastened, my arms were wet half way up to my elbows and half my back and front were also wet. Possibly if I'd put the poncho on immediately it started to rain I may have been drier.

My sister-in-law has the same coat and she'd tested it in bad weather and her coat was definitely waterproof. Maybe mine's a "Friday afternoon" one.

However, we're dry now. We're comfortably ensconced in the White Hart Inn which is fabulous. We even have a whirlpool bath! The meal this evening was very good and we enjoyed chatting to an Australian man doing the Cotswold Way.

Thursday May 18th

Leonards Stanley to Painswick **Gloucestershire** *10 miles*

We had a pleasant walk in sunny weather today with not too many hills. Unfortunately, there were no cafés. The woods were glorious and we found twayblade, a rare orchid, and star of Bethlehem, a pretty white flower, unusual to us from Lincolnshire. Also we saw a new (to us) flower called sanicle. It's a delicate white and pink flower with starry flower heads. We also saw the three-cornered leek flower again.

We diverted off the Cotswold Way to find the "Deli" that the Australian man from last night had told us about. It was never found.

We eventually arrived at the lovely old village of Painswick with its quaint, narrow streets and mellow Cotswold stone buildings, some of which were half-timbered. The churchyard had some beautiful old yew trees. We were just going into the village along a winding road when Linda slipped and fell. I was worried that a car might come round the corner but luckily it didn't. She ended up with bloody knees but bravely carried on.

We are staying at the Falcon Inn in a spacious room for three but the lighting is very poor. One light didn't go at all. The manager said he didn't have enough staff for anyone to carry our bags to our room which is over in the courtyard so we carried them ourselves. We went to a cheaper pub to eat.

Friday May 19th

Painswick to Birdlip   ***Gloucestershire***   *8 miles*

We had another hilly walk in fine weather through extensive woodlands with interesting flowers again. We saw bugle, sweet woodruff, red campion, Dame's violet and yellow archangel. There were times when the woodland opened out into buttercup meadows giving great views of Gloucester and further away we could see the Malvern Hills.

It was a disappointing day again for tea shops as at least two were promised in Linda's guide book. One was at Prinknash Abbey which we couldn't get to without going on a busy "A" road and the other café was closed. We thought Birdlip might have a café but only the pub, The George, where we are staying had cake, Bakewell tart, which we had. It wasn't bad.

We met a woman who was originally from Grimsby who's staying here and on discovering what I was doing gave me £5 for my charity.

We have lovely rooms and a bath. The staff are very friendly. We like it here. The food is good and it has a small portions menu which we all had, leaving room for large pavlovas!

Saturday May 20th

Birdlip to Woodmancote   **Gloucestershire**   *12 miles*

We reduced the walk by four miles by going off the Cotswold Way. The route is often very circuitous in order to see some historic site which we're not really bothered about as there are so many in this area. We went through fields of sheep and by farms which made a change from the usual woodlands. When we returned to the Cotswold Way it wasn't as hilly as usual which was a bonus. However, we did climb up to the highest point of the Cotswold Way which is Cleve Common at 1083 feet. It has various orchids, glow worms and many different butterflies on this large upland plateau but we didn't see many of them. We rejoined the Cotswold Way at Seven Springs, a pub with coffee and cake! Then, not long after, we

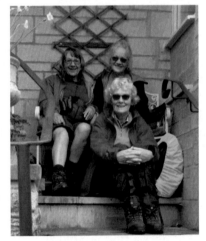

came across a cottage with an old couple who were serving drinks and toasted teacakes in the garden. We didn't like to walk by on principle so we sat on the steps enjoying our second tea break.   A group of Duke of Edinburgh boys were nearby and I told them what I was doing. They smiled and tried to look impressed.

Me, Jacky and Linda.

We saw more of the sanicle flowers today and also a tiny blue flower called chalk milkwort and yellow crosswort. We were going down a lane with hedges and fences each side when we suddenly saw a deer running towards us. On seeing us, it stopped and ran back the other way. We saw two walkers ahead, coming towards us and the deer, being in between us, was panicking. So we hid at the side. When the walkers reached us they said the deer was stuck in a hedge as it tried to escape. They asked us to go and help to free it as they noticed we had walking poles. So we all went back to where they'd seen it but it wasn't there so obviously it had freed itself and escaped. Thank goodness!

Pam, our B & B lady, met us in her car at the Golf Course on Cleeve Common and took us to her house. She drove past the pub we could go to for an evening meal but it was at least a twenty minute walk to get to from her house and we were too tired to do it. She eventually noticed the state of us and very kindly took us to a fish and chip shop and waited while we got some and then brought us back.

My little toenail is coming off and I have another blister on my big toe.

Sunday May 21st

Woodmancote to Wood Stanton **Gloucestershire**   *8 miles*

This was originally a twelve mile stretch but I cut it down to eight miles (by cutting out loops) so it was much more enjoyable. We had a self-catering continental breakfast of cereal with yoghurt, salmon, cheese, melon, fruit salad and Danish pastries. Pam had left it all in the fridge or on the table for us in our own dining area. It was delicious and a pleasant change from the normal cooked breakfast we're offered at hotels and B & B's. We took a cheese sandwich, a lemon yoghurt and a flapjack for our lunch. Pam took us back to the Golf Club House in her car to continue our walk.

It was another sunny day and the walk was not hilly. We found a café in Winchcombe and did some shopping. The village had attractive Cotswold stone houses. Unfortunately most of the shops were closed as it was a Sunday. En route we passed Hale fruit farm and had a cup of tea.

We're staying in a farmhouse that's four hundred years old at Wood Stanton. We're all in one room, Linda in the double bed and Jacky and I in bunk beds.

The lady of the house cooked us a roast chicken dinner with charred (burnt!) roast vegetables and a delicious home-made plum tart with cream. We were joined by a walker from South Africa who's now living in Holland. She's doing the Cotswold Way too but is carrying all her stuff. She said one should only carry a bag that is no more than ten per cent of your body weight. So my rucksack which weighs about 28 lbs should be about 12lbs! I've no idea what I could leave out to get it down to that.

Monday May 22nd

Wood Stanton to Chipping Campden **Gloucestershire** *11 miles*

It was a fine day today, the last day of the Cotswolds Way. I enjoyed it though it was much hillier than we thought and there were not as many teashops as we'd hoped. There were lots of groups of walkers doing The Cotswold Way, mostly doing it north to south, the opposite way to us. It's better to walk south to north as you have the sun behind you and the prevailing south westerly wind and rain behind you. They were mostly Americans and a few people from Lincolnshire. One couple we met were from Cleethorpes and had been following my progress in the Cleethorpes Chronicle. (I've been sending weekly updates to the newspaper.)

The scenery was quite different today. There were more fields of buttercups and crops, less hills and more villages.

Broadway had a lot of shops in the main street and we went to a café there. It was very warm today so we had lots of rests and drinks.

In the evening we went to the Indian restaurant within the Volunteer Inn where we are staying. Even Linda came in and had an omelette as she doesn't like Indian food. However, she said she didn't like it as it was leathery. Jacky gave me some very light navy and white spotted shoes with a sole so I can off load my trainers now. I needed them for walking around a town on a day off.

The owner of the Volunteer Inn who also does the Baggage company we've been using gave me £20 for my charity when I told him what I was doing!

Tuesday May 23rd

Chipping Campden   Day off

Linda and Jacky left in the morning. I went for a walk round the village which has very elegant and beautiful honey-coloured stone buildings and some tasteful shops down the main street. I had a cream tea in a café.

Afterwards, I looked round a very interesting museum about a man called Ashbee who was a social reformer in the East End of London at the turn of the 20th century. He decided to do the same in healthier countryside so came to Chipping Campden and set up a guild of Craftsmen, silversmiths in particular.

At lunchtime, I discovered there was a concert on in the church as luckily it was a Music Festival week in the village. I enjoyed listening to an amazing brass quintet. I realised how much I was missing live music.

Avril and her husband Mike arrived to join me again and we all went to the Silversmith workshop that Ashbee (from the museum) had set up. It was craftsmen and women making silver things and they didn't mind talking to us and showing us how they made the things. It was very interesting. There was also an art and crafts studio with things for sale.

In the evening, we all went to an Italian restaurant which was quite up market with authentic Italian food. Mike and Avril stayed at the Volunteer Inn with me. It's great to see them and know that Avril will walk with me for three days.

Wednesday May 24th

Chipping Campden to Barton (6 miles from Stratford on Avon)
Gloucestershire & Warwickshire *13 miles*

The Heart of England Way

It was very warm today. Avril and I had a lovely walk through flat and undulating countryside similar to the Lincolnshire Wolds. There were not many woods for shade. The flowers were not very interesting today apart from white campion and star of Bethlehem.

We went wrong in the middle of the day in navigation but didn't add much on in mileage. The locals we asked weren't very helpful plus I think the map I'm using is old and didn't show a Greenway track. It was very confusing.

Mike met us at the end and took us to our B & B. It has the most wonderful baby grand piano which the lady said I could play. In fact she was pleased I was playing it. There was lots of very good music in the piano stool and I also had a jazz piece that Theo had played when I stayed with Chris. She'd given me a copy of it. I really enjoyed playing the piano. It was a beautiful one.

Mike drove us to the pub at Barton for a meal. It was called "The Cottage of Content" and we found out the reason for that name. It had originally been a brothel!

Thursday May 25th

Barton to Henley- in- Arden **Warwickshire** *15 miles*

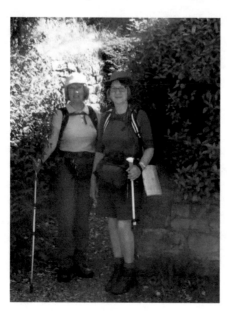

Avril joins me again

It was hot today, twenty eight degrees! It was humid. Horrendous to walk in! It was a very taxing day due to the heat and confusion over the route. Also we were chased by bullocks again and pestered by horses. At one point, we were following a footpath sign through a field of rape.

The footpath deteriorated and we had to fight our way through head-high rape, nettles and thistles, getting stung and scratched. It ended in a barbed wire fence that we had to struggle to climb.

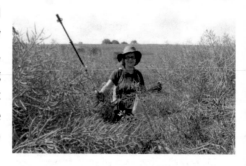

There were many high stiles too which exhausted us in the heat. Twice we went the wrong way. The GPS and compass sorted us out eventually but led to delays and extra miles.

We found a pub for a welcome coffee in the morning and sat by a river in the afternoon at Alcester for tea and cake. But mostly it was very long, hot and exhausting.

We saw white bryony flowers today. They are very pretty and wind round other plants in hedgerows. Also we saw lots of yellow crosswort and bugle.

Mike picked us up and took us to the Old Rectory which is an old, slightly dilapidated red brick building in its own grounds. It has an air of mystery. It reminded us of Bates' Hotel in Psycho!

The shower was unreliable. Avril and Mike's shower was cold but mine went warm eventually. We just ate the food Avril had bought from the shop as it was too late to go to a pub by the time we arrived. At about 11pm when I was lying in bed there was a sudden racket outside then the sound of thudding footsteps coming right up near my room. I thought people were coming in to my room. It turned out to be the family of the owner returning which we hadn't expected.

Friday May 26th

Henley- in-Arden to Balsall Common   **Warwickshire**   *10 ½ miles*

It was another hot day, twenty eight degrees but not humid. It was quite easy walking. Avril and I walked five miles along the Stratford then the Grand Union canals. We found a pub for coffee along the canal. It was very pleasant seeing colourful barges and ducklings. Then we walked through buttercup fields and a few woodlands. We had to climb one steep hill then a few small hills but mainly it was a level walk. We're staying in the Brickmakers Arms. Ian arrived by train at 8pm to spend the weekend with me.

Saturday May 27th

Balsall   Common   (Near   Coventry)   to   Nether   Whitacre
Warwickshire   *15 miles*

Avril and Mike left and they took several items from my monster bag back with them so it's now down to 23lbs which is much better. I walked with Ian and the rucksack felt OK. It was level walking with occasional small hills. It was farmland mostly with some fields with horses that fortunately didn't bother us.

We were resting beside a cottage when the owner, an old man called Dave and his dog, Meg, drove up and started chatting to us. Then he brought us out a cup of tea and a £10 donation for my charity!

Two miles west of Coventry we discovered the village of Meriden (in the West Midlands) which claims to be the centre of England. So I had a picture taken in the courtyard of the Bull's Head by the signpost.

We came off the Heart of England Way to go on some minor roads as well as some dreadfully overgrown footpaths. It was cool and cloudy weather which was much better for walking. We stopped at a village pub and rang for a taxi to take us to the Tamworth Arms (£18). We enjoyed a glass of wine and some cheese and biscuits while we were waiting. It was a very noisy pub so we sat outside. The Tamworth Arms, which is in Staffordshire, is cheap and cheerful.

Sunday May 28th

Nether Whitacre to Drayton Bassett   **Staffordshire**   *8 miles*

Ian and I had a lovely easy walk in flattish countryside and on some minor roads. We went through a water park that was extremely busy and noisy, being a Sunday. There were lots of people and also the jarring noise of jet skis and a shooting range too. There was also a little railway like the one at Cleethorpes and a café which we went to. So not very peaceful! The most interesting thing we saw were long threads hanging down from alder trees with little clumps of webs containing tiny caterpillars. People were staring at them. Some of them reached down to the ground to let the caterpillars crawl out and as you walked along you had to be careful not to bump into the long threads.

The canal banks were very attractive with yellow irises and orchids and blue damselflies. We also saw some beautiful black and blue dragonflies posing on the flowers. There were occasional meadows full of buttercups, the rare pink ragged robin and white ox-eye daisies. As we approached Drayton Basset church we saw pale pink bistort flowers and a grey wagtail.

Ian and I had a relaxing afternoon and an early evening meal prior to him catching the train back home. It was lovely to see him.

Monday May 29th

Drayton Bassett to Lichfield   **Staffordshire**   *10 miles*

I got a taxi to take me back to Drayton Bassett and I walked from the church. It was a cool and damp start. The walk through the fields and lovely woods was easy and pleasant. There were some mostly quiet roads. Then I had to go on an "A" road luckily with a footpath. It started raining quite heavily but I managed to get to a pub for a delightful lunch of a delicious cauliflower cheese tart and vegetables. The pub was very interesting with musical instruments on the walls.

The Heart of England Way goes right past Glennys' house. Glennys is a friend from school so we go back a very long way but she was also a member of my walking group until she moved to Lichfield a couple of years ago. It was lovely to see Glennys and Andrew again and they made me very welcome. Also they took me out in their car for an evening tour of Lichfield and showed me the interesting historical and literary places in the city and the magnificent Cathedral which we are hoping to visit tomorrow. The Cathedral is very impressive having three spires which is very unusual.

I carried my bag all day and now my shoulders ache. Also I lost one of my poles today, behind a hedge. I can't go back for it.

Tuesday May 30th

*Lichfield to Castle Ring **Staffordshire***   *10 miles*

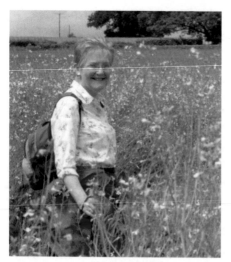

Glennys

I walked with Glennys from her house as it's on the Heart of England Way and she led me to the Cathedral where there was a Turner painting on view. It was a very interesting and beautiful Cathedral but we only had time for a short visit. I then took over the navigation and went wrong immediately. However, I soon found the right way to a park but in the park went the wrong way again and had to go through bullocks but they didn't bother us.

We retraced our steps and Andrew met us. Together, we walked through farmland, woods and wild flower meadows. There were some tall crimson clover flowers in a crop field with pea flowers and yellow rape. It was very pretty.

There were some high stiles which Glennys found tricky to climb as she has a bad hip. We arrived at a lovely pub for lunch which Andrew treated me to. Then I said goodbye to them and continued on alone with my big bag to carry again.

I walked through fields and on roads until I reached Cannock Chase at Castle Fort which is a vast forested area. I started off in the right direction then took the wrong turn due to missing the sign which was hidden in the trees. There are many footpaths in this area. I checked my compass and eventually realised I was going in the wrong direction and had to return to the start and try again! Then I met Patsy and she carried my rucksack for a mile to a lovely campsite!

Wednesday May 31st

Wandon Campsite, Rugeley to Abbots Bromley
    Staffordshire   *13 miles*

This was a day of highs and lows. Patsy lived in Rugeley for several years during World War Two to escape the bombing in Grimsby. I was not yet born then. Our father was stationed nearby and Patsy lived there with Tim, our brother, and our mother. Patsy has very fond memories of that time. She was four years old when she first went. So Patsy and I had to go on a sentimental tour of the area for her. I didn't mind. It was a beautiful sunny day.

We walked to Etchinghill and Slitting Mill to see the church where Tim had been a lamb in the Nativity Play when he was two years old. He crawled around the pews it seems! Unfortunately, the church was locked. Then we went to see the house which mum and dad rented. The house looked the worst in the row now. The school Patsy went to until she was eight years old is no longer there. We had a picnic at Etchinghill where Patsy remembers going to often as a child.

Then I continued alone while Patsy went back to the campsite. I got to a canal and walked up and down it in vain trying to find the exit path to cross the railway and get to the Staffordshire Way. After asking someone I ended up on a busy road with a footpath at the side

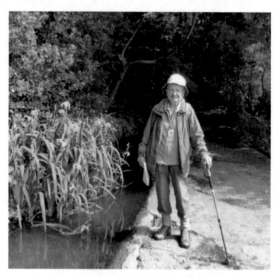

Patsy near Etchinghill, Rugeley

of it. I was quite lost and disorientated despite using the GPS and compass. Eventually I asked a woman and she showed me the way to Colton village. I found out it was a new bypass road I was on. My map was old and didn't show it!

I chatted to a lady who was planting some flowers outside a church. I told her what I was doing and that I'd had cancer three years ago so was doing the walk to celebrate my health. She took off her hat to show me her bald head. She was having chemotherapy for breast cancer.

In the same village I then met a jolly man, George, who'd also done the walk, but the other way, John O'Groats to Land's End, with his son, eight years ago. He invited me into his garden for a cup of tea and biscuits. Because I was still traumatised from getting lost, I went. We had a lovely chat and I met his wife and son. He insisted that I take a bag of mints with me when I left. I've met so many kind people!

I continued on minor roads after a cross field diversion petered out. All was going fine till I went on a footpath that began well going through lovely barley fields. I love barley fields especially when there's a breeze. It looks like the waves on the sea.

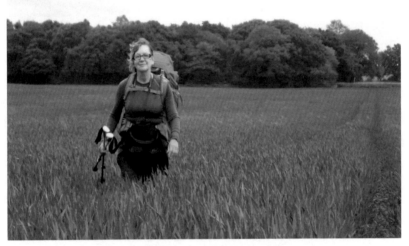

I'm walking through a barley field

There was a good view too. Then I took the wrong path to a farm. I diverted following a compass direction to pick up the correct path but the large field I was in was full of long grass and thistles. It was like wading through sand. Eventually I got to a gate which I needed to get through as there was no other way to go. However, the gate was broken. It was leaning forwards so I couldn't climb it. I couldn't undo the knot of rope that was tying up one side of it. On the other side of the gate was a chain which I also couldn't undo. I started to panic a bit and wondered whether to ring Patsy who I knew should be quite close by waiting for me on a road. She could then go to the farm ahead and ask them to come and rescue me! But I knew I shouldn't have been in that field so that was a bad idea. I had another go at the chain and luckily it came free and I got through the gate and crossed the field to the farm, hoping nobody was looking. I climbed a gate, ran across the farmyard, climbed another gate and I was in the lane. There was Patsy! What a relief! We walked back together laughing through the fields to Abbots Bromley.

Thursday June 1st

Abbots Bromley to Rocester   ***Staffordshire***   *16½   miles*
The Staffordshire Way

It was a long, tricky day today not helped by the warm, humid weather. Patsy walked with me for the first mile through fields with some cows in that ignored us. Then came a very difficult field of head-high rape that had not been cut for the path. We struggled through it using our poles to fight our way through.

I then continued alone and it was OK for a while. I sat down to have my lunch in a field and decided it was time to change the map. The new map was behind the map I was using in my map case. But when I looked I discovered to my horror that the new map was not there! I nearly panicked but decided to keep calm and think about it. I thought I would just use my compass to keep on a north east direction and follow the Staffordshire Way signs. But just in case it was my lucky day, I went back to the last stile to see if I could find it. Lo and behold there it was on the ground! What a relief! And the signs for the Staffordshire Way were few and far between so I would have really struggled without the map.

Things kept going wrong. I went the wrong way at a farm which added half a mile and then on finding the right path, I tripped as my hat had hidden a low branch from me. I fell into a bed of nettles.

As it was a warm day, my arms were bare. I stung my whole arm and the top of my leg through my trousers. Also my hand that I fell on was bruised. I went into Uttoxeter and found a chemist. I bought some sting relief cream and smothered it on my arm. Then I went in a café to recover with tea and cake.

After that, I went the wrong way again for a mile trying to find the Staffordshire Way. It's certainly not well signed. I couldn't find the exit in a field of cows and bullocks so continued until I could climb over a fence into the next field.

I decided to go to Doveridge village instead and use minor roads. That added another two miles. I braved another field of cows and bullocks that actually ran away from me. It led me to a footpath and then some road walking. By now, I was totally exhausted.

I met Patsy on the road and on reaching the camper van we went on a long drive to get to our new campsite at Overton. The lady there, Mrs Bloor, gave us the £12 fee back when she heard what I was doing for my charity.

Friday June 2nd

Rocester to Tissington   **Staffordshire and Derbyshire**   *12 miles*

The Limestone Way

It was another difficult day but lovely too. The weather was cool but still humid. There were now hills and great views and many buttercups fields with clover, delicate white pignut and ox-eye daisies too. Many stiles, often tricky narrow ones with holly growing next to them made life difficult. Squeeze stiles too were not easy and I'm not even fat, in fact I'm getting thinner with all this excessive exercise! There were several fields of cows and bullocks. I was very brave walking through one and none bothered me. I deserve a medal for going through one field that had a large bull in

71

it sitting with its harem of cows and calves round it. I had to walk past them on the path about five yards away and they ignored me but I was very nervous.

It was a long day with slow progress through grassy fields and up hills. The signs for the Limestone Way were not distinguishable from other footpath signs. I did some good navigation and didn't get lost once.

There was a very heavy rain shower in the afternoon. I was in a large field of sheep and I sheltered under some trees while it poured down. Some of the sheep were under trees but I noticed that others that were in the open stood like statues with their backs slightly humped. I felt guilty that I was under the trees that they should have been sheltering under but on moving off, when the rain eased a bit, they still remained like statues. It was very strange. I finished my walk on the Tissington Trail walking fast after trudging for quite a while.

Saturday June 3rd

Tissington to Streethead Farm, Pomeroy   **Derbyshire**   *13 miles*

The Pennine Bridleway

Carole, my friend who plays in the Whitfield Guitar group with Ian and me, drove up from Cleethorpes to walk with me for two days. It was great to see her. She's also in my walking group so is quite a good walker but doesn't walk regularly as she works full time.

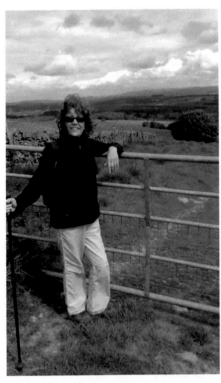

Carole

It was a fine, cool and breezy day as we walked the easy route along the straight and flat Tissington Trail. We were pleased to see a café along there and I queued up to get us a coffee. In front of me was an older man who offered the assistant a £50 note for two teas and a flapjack. This was refused and he opened his wallet to reveal a wad of £50 notes saying that was all he had. He turned to me, smiling, saying he'd just printed them that morning! They said he could have the teas for nothing but not the flapjack. I offered to buy him the flapjack but he said he couldn't possibly let me. As Carole and I were sitting outside drinking our coffees he passed by and thanked me for offering to pay. I told him that I'd received many kindnesses in the last few weeks and wanted to do the same for someone else. Then I told him about my walk and my charity for the Duke of Edinburgh Award Scheme for disadvantaged youngsters in our area. With that, he delved into his pocket and gave me one of the £50 notes. What a wonderful gesture!

Carole and I then went along the Pennine Bridleway to our campsite. Carole set up her large tent. It was lovely and so roomy!

Then we went with Patsy to the pub for our evening meal. The route was across two fields, one with bullocks that ignored us. Then we had to climb up onto a high stile which Patsy, who is almost eighty, did easily and then stood on the top without holding on. My heart was in my mouth! She is intrepid! There then followed a series of steep, rocky, uneven steps to climb down (and back up later). Carole and I were slow and cautious. Patsy was like a mountain goat! We had a good evening at the pub.

Sunday June 4th

Streethouse Farm, Pomeroy to 2 miles east of Chapel en le Frith
Derbyshire   *16 miles*

Patsy walked with Carole and I for about a mile over three fields with difficult stiles then went back to the campsite. The Pennine Bridleway was mostly good for fast walking. Occasionally, it went on minor roads. We arrived at Miller's Dale and had a drink in the lovely old pub there. Then we decided to go through Monks Dale which we'd never been to before. It was a lush, beautiful wood. There were ferns and orchids as well as other wild flowers: water avens, crosswort and possibly star of Bethlehem. However, it was very slow going. The path was narrow, rocky and overgrown and in places there were fallen trees which we had to climb over. I was just telling Carole that I was glad she was with me as if I stumbled and lay injured it might be days before anyone found me when there appeared a stream of people! There were families with children carrying their bikes as the terrain was impossible to get through on a bike if you were trying to ride it. There were Sunday strollers out for a bit of an adventure.

Then suddenly we saw two men coming towards us with a huge dog. One of the men was wearing a bright yellow vest which said John O'Groats to Land's End for Cancer research.

I hailed him with excitement saying that I was doing the same walk but the other way. He told me he'd started it with his wife but she'd had to stop and go home because of an injured foot. He introduced the other guy who he had met by chance who was also doing the same walk with his dog. What a coincidence! I don't know if they were just together for that day or had decided to continue together. Because of the narrowness of the path and people wanting to get past, we could only chat together briefly but they did say they'd met another lady who was doing LeJog too.

We only did a couple of miles through Monks Dale because we were making such slow progress. We returned to the Pennine Bridleway. Then it started to rain, and we went the wrong way adding extra miles. There was also a hill at the end too but we didn't feel too exhausted as it had been cool and there were no stiles to climb except at the beginning. Carole did well. She drove back home after a bite to eat.

Monday June 5th

A road 2 miles east of Chapel en le Frith to Broadbottom Station
***Derbyshire/Greater Manchester** 13 miles*

It was wet and windy all day today. I was walking on my own on the Pennine Bridleway which was quite a good route, usually on tracks or lanes with no fields to cross. I did vary it a bit however when there was a field with cows and bullocks in. I detoured to avoid them by going to a farm but then had to climb a wall to get out onto a road. I went to a pub at Hayfield for soup and a coffee. I went on a few minor roads.

At first, I climbed quite high on the Pennine Bridleway and despite the rain I enjoyed the views across to the dark brooding splendour of Kinderscout. I could see the Downfall in the distance where the family and I put Alex's ashes in 2002. (Alex was my second husband.

He died of a heart attack.) We have been on pilgrimages there several times but the last time was last year when I climbed it alone. Usually it's been weather like today up on the mountain: rainy, misty and windy. But last year I went up in glorious sunshine and had fabulous views for a change. It was a hilly walk today in places but I enjoyed it despite the weather.

Patsy met me and we drove to our new campsite. It's in a high, bleak car park and it's very wet and windy here. The wind is whistling. So Patsy is sleeping in the camper van with me. We went for our evening meal to the hotel 100 yards away and enjoyed it. We were told that there was a couple staying here who are also doing LeJog but we haven't seen them.

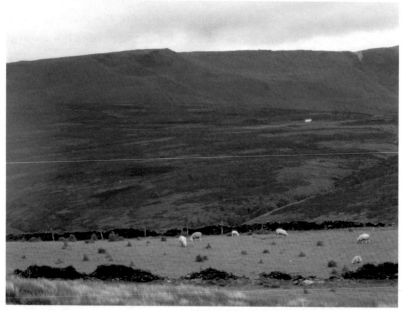

Kinderscout with Kinder Downfall on the right on the horizon

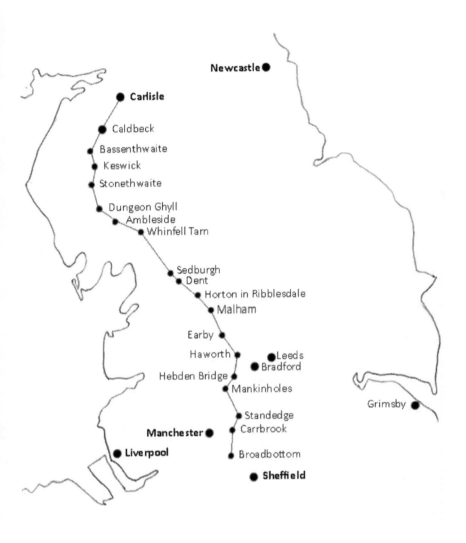

Newcastle ●

● Carlisle

● Caldbeck

Bassenthwaite
● Keswick
● Stonethwaite

● Dungeon Ghyll
● Ambleside
● Whinfell Tarn

● Sedburgh
● Dent
● Horton in Ribblesdale
● Malham

Earby ●
Haworth ● ● Leeds
Hebden Bridge ● ● Bradford
● Mankinholes

● Standedge
Manchester ● ● Carrbrook
● Liverpool
● Broadbottom

● Sheffield

Grimsby ●

Stage 3

Broadbottom to Carlisle

77

Stage 3 Broadbottom to Carlisle   6/6 – 23/6

		Ordinance Survey Map
Broadbottom to Carrbrook	10 miles	Ex. OL1
Standedge to Mankinholes	17 miles	Ex. OL21
Mankinholes to Haworth	15 miles	Ex. OL21
Haworth to Earby	15 miles	Ex. OL21
Earby to Malham (Gordale Scar)	15 miles	Ex. OL21 & Ex. OL2
Malham to Horton in Ribblesdale	13 miles	Ex. OL2
Horton in Ribblesdale to Dent	16 miles	Ex. OL2
Dent to Sedburgh	7 miles	Ex. OL19
Sedburgh to Whinfell Tarn	13 miles	Ex. OL19 & Ex. OL7
Whinfell Tarn to Ings	10 miles	Ex. OL7
Ings to Ambleside	10 miles	Ex. OL7
Ambleside to Dungeon Ghyll	8 miles	Ex. OL7 & Ex. OL6
Dungeon Ghyll to Stonethwaite	9 miles	Ex. OL6 & Ex. OL4
Stonethwaite to Keswick	9 miles	Ex. OL4
Keswick to Bassenthwaite	12 ½ miles	Ex. OL4
Bassenthwaite to Caldbeck	10 ½ miles	Ex. OL4 & Ex. OL5
Caldbeck to Carlisle	15 miles	Ex. OL5 & Ex.315
Carlisle	Day off	**Total 205 miles**

17 walking days. Average 12 miles per day. Days off: 1

Tuesday June 6th

Broadbottom to Carrbrook

Greater Manchester/West Yorkshire   *10 miles*

The Trans Pennine Trail

The Pennine Bridleway

A very difficult day today due to rain and gales and going the wrong way at times.

I started off going the wrong way down the Trans Pennine trail and had to start again. Very frustrating but I hadn't gone far. One part was very lovely near a Nature Reserve. There were beautiful trees and the grassy path was undulating. But then I went the wrong way and ended up in a cow field where they all followed me. I couldn't see the exit so walked as quickly as I could to the nearest fence which I had thought was a gate. I jumped over it pretty smartly as a cow was directly behind me!

I enjoyed watching an aerial display from three curlews calling to each other. The sound of curlews brings back memories of my father who used to call us by whistling like a curlew. (I know....like the poor children of Captain Von Trapp in The Sound of Music who responded to their father's whistles!) However, I discovered that curlews have many different calls, not just the one that we grew up with. I also saw a weasel darting across the path.

Later I came across the sign that you never want to see...."path closed". This can lead to extra miles if you try to go a different way so it's always best to try to negotiate the difficulty if at all possible. So I went to see what the problem was. I discovered it was a broken bridge over a stream. I went along the stream and jumped across it at the narrowest point then went under the orange netting that had been put up as a barrier. No problem!

Eventually, I got on the Pennine Bridleway path and went on it the wrong way. I had to go back on it again the correct way. I'd inadvertently walked in a circle. I walked past reservoirs and then cut across a hill to speed up my progress but I shouldn't have bothered. It was so windy it made the going very difficult and slow.

At 6pm, I was exhausted and decided I'd had enough and could go no further. I was on the edge of a town and I knew Patsy was waiting for me at Standedge, six miles away. She probably had no signal and would have got hopelessly lost trying to find me so I decided it would be best to call a taxi. Of course I didn't know the number of a taxi but I thought if I waited a while somebody might come along that I could ask. Sure enough a man came out with his dog. I asked him if he knew the number of a taxi and he did. So I rang the taxi and was taken up to bleak Standedge Edge where Patsy was waiting in the camper van. I was chilled through. The heater in the camper van refuses to come on for some unknown reason. So we can't dry my clothes.

Wednesday June 7th

Standedge to Mankinholes   **West Yorkshire**   *17 miles*

The Pennine Way

Zoë, my daughter, rang this morning. Nico and Gabriel, the two year old twins, have got chicken pox. She said how much all the boys are enjoying the Squeaky emails and the postcards. Kyriacos is seven now and Alexander is four. Ever since Kyriacos, my first grandson, was born, I've taken a pink mouse puppet called Squeaky to see them when I go to London. I told them that Squeaky is on this adventure with me and every week I send them emails and photos

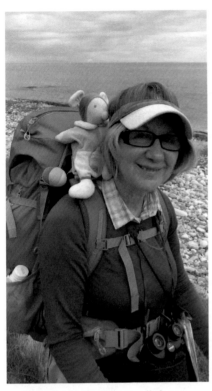
Squeaky was with me all the way

of what Squeaky has been up to, as well as sending them postcards of where we are. I'm glad they're enjoying them.

Patsy walked with me for about a mile then went back as she was going home today. I am now on the Pennine Way which I have joined here at Standedge and will do just 75 miles of it. The whole route is 267 miles long. As I have done the Pennine Way before I didn't want to do it all as I know it's mostly moors and bogs and very bleak. However, because it is situated in the middle of the country going from south to north it's an obvious choice of route for people walking LeJog. I decided to use the Pennine Bridleway at first and just join the Pennine Way here. A good idea possibly though not without its difficulties.

It was very windy and cold along the bleak moorland path but the myriad dancing cottongrass and the waving rushes softened the scene. After a while, I realised I was going in the wrong direction so retraced my steps but it only added on half a mile, so not too bad. Again, I enjoyed watching a curlew displaying and calling.

I was walking along a reservoir when I came across the dreaded "path closed" sign. I looked on my map and decided to divert across some fields to the Rochdale Canal. This was a lovely flat straight path which was very pleasant for a few miles. However by the time I'd reached the canal I was worn out.

I walked along some minor roads and arrived at the Youth Hostel at 8.30pm! I knew it was a self-catering hostel and Patsy had given me a tin of spaghetti Bolognese and some fruit. I also had some delicious chocolate cake that my friend, Jan, from my walking group had sent me via her brother. She was due to walk with me today but wasn't able to come as her husband was ill. So she'd sent her brother, who lives near here, to meet me this morning at Standedge with the cake that his wife had made. It was absolutely delicious. I think Jan was very lucky not to have had the exhausting and difficult day I've had today although of course together, it would have been much better.

Thursday June 8th

Mankinholes to Haworth   **West Yorkshire**   *15 miles*

I quite enjoyed the walk to Hebden Bridge despite the light rain. It's a very attractive place with the Rochdale canal running through it and several interesting bridges. There are some lovely shops and it's a centre for artists and creative people. I would have liked to have stayed longer. In Hebden Bridge, I found a nice café and had cake and coffee. I then wandered around, basically looking for the way out to go towards Haworth. Eventually I went to the Tourist Information Office who gave me a map to get to Hardcastle Crags which I discovered is marked on the map too far to the west which was a great confusion. I walked through hilly woodland. By 3.30pm, I'd arrived at a minor road and decided to send my heavy rucksack ahead in a taxi to the B & B in Haworth.

The weather deteriorated with many heavy showers interspersed with short bursts of sunshine to lull me into taking off some layers just before the next heavy shower soaked me. I went over Penistone Hill hoping to see the poems on the rocks that I remembered from another time I'd been here but I must have gone a different way as I missed them. I saw a water vole scuttle across the path and also enjoyed the curlews and lapwings.

The paths were very stony and had turned into streams. It was hilly and my progress was slow and difficult.

Eventually, I arrived at the lovely pristine B & B at Haworth at 8pm. The owner told me the pub that was 100 yards away finished serving food at 8.30pm. Despite being exhausted and looking like a drowned rat, I managed to have the quickest shower and hair wash and was at that bar by 8.25pm! The barmaid told me that they actually served food till 9.30pm!

There was only one other person, a middle aged man, in the lounge. I ate my meal with a glass of wine and wrote an email to my friend. I told her how depressed and lonely I was feeling and what awful weather I'd been having and how exhausted I was. Suddenly, I found I was crying. Not only crying but sobbing loudly! The man came over and asked if I was alright. So I sobbed out how I was feeling and told him about my walk and that I couldn't give up as all these people were supporting me and sponsoring me. After talking with him and drinking the second glass of wine that he bought me, I started to feel better. Quite tipsy actually! But how embarrassing!

That night, I felt unwell and the next morning had a stomach upset. So whether the mental state caused the upset tum or the other way round I don't know.

Friday June 9th

Haworth to Earby   ***West Yorkshire and Lancashire***   *15 miles*

The Pennine Way

This was another very long, hard day, not helped by the depression I was feeling and the delicate tummy I had. I set off without any breakfast as I didn't think it wise to eat anything after my tummy upset. I took some tablets. I sent my bag ahead in a taxi. I had no energy but thought I should make an effort as if I took a day off, it would disrupt all the accommodation plans for the future. However, after a couple of miles, I came across a pub that was open so I had a cranberry juice and some salted peanuts. I started to feel better as I walked up onto the moors on the Pennine Way.

It was quite pleasant, sunny with a cool breeze. First thing this morning, at Haworth, there was a shower but no rain after that. On top of the moors, I found a small semi-circular stone wall shelter, possibly for sheep. It seemed the perfect place for my lunch. I thought I'd better have a wee first and had a good 360 degree look round. No one in sight at all. I was just starting to take my trousers down when I heard a man's voice shouting out "Ahoy there!" Suddenly three men appeared from a dip. "We're the three musketeers!" they called out to me and we all laughed as I quickly pulled up my trousers. What a surprise! Then the views opened out and it was glorious. There was heather in bud and I made fast progress along the stone slabs but often there was the usual mud, bogs, rocks and pools to negotiate round.

Once I got off the moors, I went on a minor road. It was nice to meet a young local couple who said they would support me online. I also met two men on the Pennine Way who chatted. Eventually, I went on the Pendle Way which was pleasant to start with. It also went through some cow and bullock fields; one lot did approach me

84

but it wasn't too bad. It took ages to reach Ian who was meeting me for the weekend near Earby. I didn't reach him till 8.30pm so we found the nearest pub and had a meal there then walked back to our B & B at Earby which wasn't far away. It was lovely to see Ian again.

Saturday June 10th

Earby to Malham (Gordale Scar) **North Yorkshire**   *5 miles*

I had a surprisingly good day today after the long dreary days I've been experiencing. It was helped by being with Ian. It's so much better to have a companion to walk with. The bad weather and trials I face on many days don't seem so bad when there's someone to share them with. It also helped that I sent the bag ahead in a taxi again. There was no high level walking either.

The scenery was lovely. We went on the Pennine Way but also on some other footpaths and minor roads. We found two cafés too! The walk towards Gordale Scar along the river valley was exceptionally wonderful. Even though it was raining, it was very beautiful along the Malham Beck which was in full spate. There were trees that had fallen in the river, rocky cliff sides to walk beside and the aroma of ramsons, wild garlic. The walk finished at Janet's Foss with the spectacular waterfall and magical grotto. It's reputed in local folklore to be the home of Jennet, the Queen of the Fairies who lived in a cave near the waterfall. (See the picture on the back cover.)

Ian and I set up the tent at Gordale Scar campsite which is a very basic campsite used almost exclusively by Duke of Edinburgh's Award youngsters. I was given special permission to camp there free of charge when I told the farmer I was doing my walk for that charity. He was delighted and said I could camp there any time I liked. As I hate camping I won't be taking him up on that offer but he was very kind. I donated the fee of £4.50 to the charity.

I saw lots of D of E youngsters who were exhausted from their treks and chatted to them in the very scruffy toilet and wash room. There were no showers. I enjoyed the camping better than usual as Ian had bought a slightly bigger tent with a double skin so that when you touch the sides of the tent from the inside you don't get wet.

After setting up camp, we walked up a steep minor road to Malham village and met Rachel my step daughter and her husband Jorge and daughter Chenoa. It was great to see them. We all enjoyed a delicious meal in the pub. And luckily they drove us back to the campsite.

Sunday June 11th

Malham (Gordale Scar) to Horton in Ribblesdale

North Yorkshire   *13 miles*

The Ribble Way

I slept quite well considering I was in my least favourite accommodation, a tent. Ian made us some of his delicious porridge for breakfast and we ate it while surveying the wonderful scenery surrounding us. Gordale Scar is a limestone ravine. It has two waterfalls and overhanging limestone cliffs that are 100 metres high. We were camping in a field by the river and to view the limestone cliffs and spectacular waterfalls of Gordale Scar, you have to walk about 200 yards and go round a corner so they were not visible from the tent.

Ian was navigating today to give me a break and he hasn't been here before. I asked him which way we were going and he indicated vaguely towards the Scar area. He didn't go into detail but I thought he probably knew what he was doing. However, as we approached the corner towards the Scar, I started to worry. On asking him where exactly the path was that we were going to take, he said it was round the corner. Oh no! I knew that there was a path that goes up by the waterfall. It's very steep and dangerous and exceedingly difficult!

In fact, many years ago, my sister Patsy took my son Nick and his cousin Steve, when they were about 10 years old, for a walk around here. When they saw the huge cliff of Gordale Scar, they were keen to climb it. Patsy said they could climb up to a certain point and then they must promise to come back down. Of course they were so excited to be climbing up the rocky waterfall that they just kept going till they got to the top.

By this time, they were completely out of sight and the noise of the waterfall had drowned out Patsy's calls to them to come back. After waiting in vain for them to return, she decided to make her way back on other paths to get back to the Youth Hostel where they were all staying at Malham. There was no sign of the boys. She was so worried about them that she called the Mountain Rescue out. Eventually, the boys found their way back and were told off by Patsy and the Mountain Rescue Team! You see even at that tender age they both had the family adventure gene!

So when Ian looked at the precipitous climb ahead he realised, thank goodness, that it wasn't a safe thing to do, especially carrying big rucksacks. So we went on a different, longer route to climb out of the valley, but gentler and much safer. There were grassy moors on either side of the paths and hilly minor roads. Eventually, we came across a pub for a cup of tea and we were in luck as a lady had brought in some home-made banana and cinnamon cakes which she was giving out free to customers to celebrate her birthday!

We then went on the Ribble Way which was a narrow footpath along a river. It was flooded at times and made my boots wet inside. There were views of Pen-y-ghent and Ingleborough, two of the three peaks which Ian has climbed several times. We eventually arrived at the Crown Inn at Horton in Ribblesdale where my friend Linda was already waiting.

Ian had to leave without a meal as his train was at 6.30pm and there was no time to eat. Linda and I had a nice meal and I sorted my bag out and had a lovely bath. It was great to see Linda again as I hadn't seen her since the Cotswold Way. She's going to walk part of the Dales Way with me for five days.

Monday June 12th

Horton in Ribblesdale to Dent   **North Yorkshire and Cumbria**
       16 miles

Linda and I walked well to start with and we had no problems finding the way. That is until we tried to find the Ribble Way. There was a signpost which had four signs pointing out the different directions possible. However, on the ground there were only three obvious paths. The Ribble Way appeared to go in between two of the signs up a hill. We tried that way but decided it didn't seem right. We decided to try one of the more obvious tracks though I wasn't convinced it was the right way. After 200 yards, I did another compass and map check and decided it was definitely over a boggy looking stretch of moorland and over a hill. I was sure it would definitely take us to the Ribble Way. Linda was not convinced. She followed me very reluctantly, sure I was taking her to a certain death by sinking into the bog. It was quite tricky fighting our way through the rushes, mud and boggy ground but we got there. On a gate was a clear sign – "The Ribble Way". If only there had been better signs before!

Eventually, we crossed a bridge to a road which led to the Dales Way. The narrow path was still muddy and boggy across the moors. However, we were overjoyed to see a sign advertising teas outside a solitary cottage! I knocked on the door but despite a light shining through the window, nobody came. How disappointing! In fact, we thought it was a cruel trick and that the owner should at least remove the sign if she had to go out. But, undaunted, (though unrefreshed), we had to go on.

The last part of our walk was along the minor road past Dent viaduct which is very impressive. It has 10 arches and is 100 feet high and 199 yards long. It's made of massive blocks of Dent marble. It was built in the late 19th century. If you're very lucky you can see a steam train crossing it but we didn't see one today.

We eventually reached the charming quaint old village of Dent at 7.15pm after a tiring day. We're now in the lovely, comfortable George Inn in the centre of Dent by the cobbled village centre.

Tuesday June 13th

Dent to Sedburgh   **Cumbria**   *7 miles*

The Dales Way

At last I had a day of easy walking along the Dales Way with Linda. We started off by exploring the interesting little shops in the village. I bought a purple merino woollen hat from a specialist knitting shop. It was in a basket with other things, one of which I noticed was £12. It was quite expensive I thought but I'd buy it. I proffered a £20 note to the lady. She waited, looking at me and I waited for my change, looking at her. Eventually she told me it was actually £30! However she said I could have it for £25. Linda encouraged me to get it as a lasting and beautiful memento of my walk. So I got it. Just hope I never lose it!

We enjoyed walking along the river looking at pale pink bistort flowers, purple tufted vetch and the pink lacy flowers of ragged robin. We noticed that the first meadow sweet was out. It's one my favourite flowers. Its creamy froth of flower heads has a lovely sweet aroma. It was my mother's favourite flower too. As we walked along, we could see the beautiful smooth Howgill Hills wreathed in mist. They always remind me of elephant backs.

We went through a lovely hamlet, Milthrop. On arrival in Sedbergh, which is a small market town, we enjoyed a cream tea in a very interesting café that sold all sorts of handmade knick-knacks. I managed not to buy any. We bought some food for tomorrow night's meal when we know we won't have any restaurant or pub nearby. We're staying in a delightful old cottage with a very old and feisty lady owner who used to live in Australia as a child. She proudly told us that she was 90 years old. It was like being in your granny's house. It was very homely and old fashioned but quirky too. There was a door to open to go up the winding stairs and the ceiling and walls were sloping. At one point she had to go out to the shops and she left the door unlocked. A man walked in with a newspaper for her then a woman walked in who'd come to walk the dog for her. It was all very interesting and heart-warming in a way. It felt like we were living in another age where life was more innocent and safe.

Wednesday June 14th

Sedbergh to Whinfell Tarn   **Cumbria**   *13 miles*

We had a good day today walking in sunny weather. We started off on undulating minor roads for four miles then joined the Dales Way again. We had to climb a gate to start with as the stile looked unusable. It was a difficult path to start with and we weren't quite sure if we really were on the Dales Way but eventually it was OK. We had lunch in a meadow with lovely views of the Howgills.

We passed by the beautiful modern bungalow, Morland Barn, that we have stayed in before but this year it was full so we had to book the only B & B we found near here which is a mile north of the Dales Way and has no food. (Hence the buying of food in Sedbergh for tonight). I left my walking pole twice today, each time we stopped, and had to go back a quarter of a mile each time for it! Linda says I've got two yellow cards for leaving it but I told her that as she is the pole monitor in our walking group, she needs a red card!

We walked to Crook Howe B & B which is by a lovely lake, Whinfell Tarn. The B & B is much bigger and better than we'd imagined and the lady is very pleasant. We ate the salad, salmon and eggs we'd bought at Sedbergh and had a nice pudding of apricots and chocolate.

My brother Tim and Chris his wife then arrived as they are camping near Ambleside. They brought us some strawberries from their garden so we had extra dessert. Delicious! We sat by the tarn (lake) chatting and arranged to walk with them tomorrow. It was a lovely evening and we enjoyed watching swans and their cygnets on the lake.

Thursday June 15th

Whinfell Tarn to Ings   **Cumbria**   *10 miles*

Linda and I walked with Tim and Chris from our B & B. Tim walked just a few miles with us and then went back to pick up his camper van. So Chris, Linda and I continued along the Dales Way to Stavely where Linda and I found a café and said goodbye to Chris. Then we cut off about three miles of our intended route by going on a main road with a footpath alongside it. Our accommodation at Ings is a Brewery/Pub. It's quite modern and very busy but comfortable enough with good food too.

Friday June 16th

Ings to Ambleside **Cumbria** *10 miles*

Linda and I had an adventure today! We started off walking along minor roads and then along a footpath going over fields on the Dales Way. The route then led to a bridge which we had to cross over a wide rushing stream. However the bridge was broken, on its side. It's not a good idea to go on a diversion or go back as it can add miles on to your day.

So, being stalwart members of the Lincolnshire Ladies Adventure Group, we climbed up onto the stone buttress and crawled across the wooden planks of the bridge! It was a bit scary, looking down into the rushing water but we kept focussed on the end of the bridge and climbed down safely.

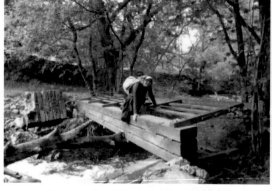

I'm crawling over a broken bridge.

We took the wrong path after a while but saw some lovely waterfalls. We eventually arrived at a locked gate and checked the GPS. We were in the wrong place. A runner luckily came along and showed us the right way. We went through a lovely wooded area leading down to Ambleside. The views would have been good from our high position over Lake Windermere but it was misty over the mountains and the lake.

The wild flowers we've seen over the last two days are tormentil, that tiny yellow flower with four petals and the yellow and orange mimulus or monkey flower that grows in streams round here. We saw common valerian in bud and yellow poppies, foxgloves and an unknown little white flower. We also spotted the unusual tall, delicate, bell-like flower that we saw in the woods in the Cotswolds. I have found out what is. It's a rare garden escape called fringecups that has now naturalised.

We're staying at Ambleside Youth Hostel which is a large, modern Hostel overlooking Lake Windermere. We are in a private room with two bunk beds for the extortionate price of £89 but there was no other accommodation to be had anywhere in this very popular place. We had fish and chips outside, looking over the lake.

Saturday June 17th

Ambleside to Dungeon Ghyll   **Cumbria**   *8 miles*

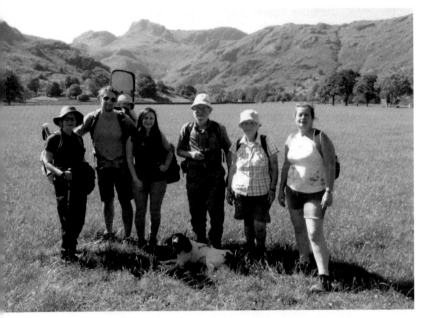

Me, Andy with baby Isla, Jenny, my brother Tim, Chris, Rachel and Boris the dog in Langdale.

Today was meant to be my day off but Avril, who is walking with me tomorrow, suggested it would be a good idea if I did eight miles today so as to reduce the distance tomorrow when we have a hard climb up Stake Pass. Good idea! Also, unexpectedly, some of my family walked with me today. It was so good to see them.

I met my brother Tim and sister-in-law Chris in Ambleside. We were joined by their son Andy and his wife Jenny and baby Isla and their dog Boris. My stepdaughter Rachel also came to walk with us. We had a lovely walk through Langdale. It was very hot but we were OK as it was not too hilly and we had two pub stops and an ice cream too. There were wonderful views of the Langdale Pikes and Crinkle Crags. However, we felt sorry for the hundreds of people walking past us the other way who were walking 26 miles on a charity walk! Some were wearing unsuitable clothing and footwear and most looked exhausted! I do think it's wrong to encourage people who may only have walked along the promenade at Cleethorpes before to nearly kill themselves on these charity walks. It will probably put them off walking for life! They would get just as much money for charity if they asked them to do a more reasonable mileage like 10 miles.

Avril and her husband Mike came to fetch us in their car from Tim's campsite and took Rachel and I back to Ambleside. We ate at the Youth Hostel Bistro and the food was surprisingly good. However, I'm now on the top bunk in a dormitory and my hand is hurting. It is swollen from the fall in the nettles that happened two weeks ago. I'm on anti-histamines. It hurts when I try to open a gate or put weight on it. It was tricky climbing up to this top bunk but all the other bunks were taken.

Sunday June 18th

Dungeon Ghyll to Stonethwaite   ***Cumbria***   *9 miles*

The Cumbria Way

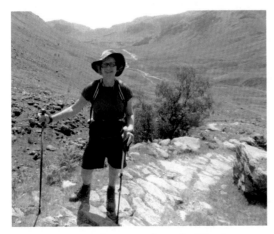

Climbing up Stake Pass, The Lake District

I had a lovely day today. It was very hot. Mike took Avril and me in the car to Tim's campsite at Dungeon Ghyll and he walked with us to the start of the trail. Avril and I were worried about climbing Stake Pass in the heat but it was OK. We started by walking along Mickledon on the Cumbria Way and there were wonderful clear views of mountains all around us. Then we had the rocky climb up Stake Pass.

It was not as hard as we remembered, from a few years ago, probably because we are both much fitter now. At the top, we met a pleasant American couple who took our pictures.

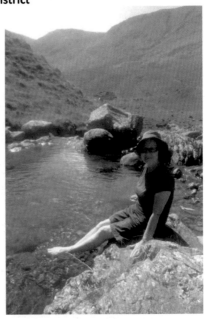

A wonderful cold dip

There was a steep zigzag path down into Langstrath Vale that is featured at the beginning of the Countryfile TV show.

It's magnificent!

We rested at the bottom and dipped our feet in the cold rock pool of the river that runs through the valley. Lovely!

We met a group of ladies who were doing the Cumbria Way and one of them gave me a £2 donation. Eventually, we arrived at our B & B in Stonethwaite. It's a lovely old cottage, Knottsview, with a delightful garden that has red squirrels in it! We saw them feeding on a bird feeder! Also we saw a great spotted woodpecker and siskins! The pub is a few yards away and we enjoyed a delicious meal there. However, there is no signal and no T.V. here. You can't have everything. So we did crosswords. Avril helped me with the clues that Linda and I had struggled with.

Monday June 19th

Stonethwaite to Keswick **Cumbria** *9 miles*

It was another lovely day, warm weather but easy walking along Borrowdale to Keswick along the river Derwent. We saw the pink betony flower. We passed Castle Crag and I would have liked to climb it but Avril wasn't keen and so we didn't. It did look rather high and it was too hot today anyway. There was lots of shade through the woods along the river to Derwent Water. I bought another poncho, bright pink as I think the camouflage one I have at the moment is dangerous as drivers struggle to see me if I'm walking along a road in dismal weather. However, I've decided it's too small and I will need to change it tomorrow. We're staying in a lovely hotel, The Keswick Park. We had a very good meal. They specialise in fish. In fact, I think it's the best accommodation I've been in so far.

Tuesday June 20th

Keswick to Bassenthwaite   **Cumbria**   *12 ½ miles*

I had another great day today with continued warm weather. I walked up and round the side of Skiddaw with Avril. There was a scarily narrow path at times with sheer drops to one side! We met two cyclists, Jeff and Keith, who gave me £10 each for my charity after we chatted to them about what I was doing. People are so kind. It was hard enough for us to walk along the path so I've no idea how cyclists manage to do it. I think they sometimes must have to walk with their bikes.

The walk was going well until we came across another bridge that was down and we couldn't get round it because the builders had put high fences and scaffolding up. It was only half a mile away from our farmhouse destination, High Side Farm. So we diverted across field paths to the village of Bassenthwaite and luckily the pub was open! So despite it only being 5pm we ate a meal there before continuing another mile across the fields to our farmhouse. There are lots of flies here but the rooms are large and luxurious. However, I can't work the TV.

Wednesday June 21st

Bassenthwaite to Caldbeck   **Cumbria**   *10 ½ miles*

There was one heavy shower as we were having breakfast but otherwise it was another very warm and humid day. We had to use alternative footpaths to go from High Side Farm to avoid the broken bridge that we encountered on our way here. This involved a steep, muddy and precipitous woodland descent to a bridge across a river and then some fields. We did some walking on minor roads which were mostly the Cumbria Way. We also went on grassy tracks at the side of the fells. The fells are getting less and less now. It's mainly undulating paths and roads. The flowers we saw today were common valerian, tufted vetch, bird's foot trefoil and mimulus (monkey flower).

As we were walking along, we met a local man with a dog (not on a lead). The dog ran ahead of us and chased some sheep quite aggressively. I asked him if he was not worried that his dog might be shot for worrying the sheep. We've come across several notices pinned on gates to that effect. He said he lived next door to the farmer and appeared not at all sorry or worried about his dog's behaviour. Amazing! We rescued some sheep that had escaped from a field and were running down the road. They went into a field where the gate was open so we shut it quickly and went to the nearest farm and told someone. At Caldbeck, we had tea and cake in a café and chatted to an Irish couple.

We're staying at the Oddfellows Arms which is not bad.

Thursday June 22nd

Caldbeck to Carlisle   **Cumbria**   *15 miles*

It was a cooler, fresher day today as Avril and I walked happily along. It was a quite easy, undulating path along the river and through woods and fields. We saw betony flowers, marsh woundwort, St John's wort, mimulus and lots of common spotted orchids in the woods. The most beautiful and unusual flower that we saw in the woods was a white and mauve climbing plant that I have identified as wood vetch. A surprisingly pretty white umbellifer flower I have discovered today is the ground elder that no one wants in their garden as it is very invasive. It certainly looks very attractive along the river banks.

We had quite an interesting encounter with a heron. We think we startled it as we suddenly saw it lifting off and flying away making a terrible sound that neither of us had ever heard a heron make before. We think that we actually saved a female goosander and her chicks from it as they were very near to where it happened. We also saw buzzards, a kestrel and oystercatchers. Sand martins were swooping along in and out of the river bank.

Our taste buds were rewarded by finding a café in a village four miles from Carlisle. We enjoyed a cream tea there. This sustained us along a long, boring tarmac path by a river into Carlisle. Our B & B is clean and cheap; The Cornerhouse. However, I'm in the attic room where my shower is down a flight of stairs. The shower would go either hot or cold but not just warm. I couldn't get the door to lock to my room either. After many phone calls (as no one actually lives here), a girl came and demonstrated that you have to slam the door to make it close properly!

Avril, Mike and I went to Wetherspoons for a nice curry and a glass of wine. I sorted out my bag and Avril is taking a few things home with her to make it a bit lighter.

Friday June 23rd

Carlisle Day off

Despite the horrible little room and problems with the shower, they managed to cook a decent breakfast at The Cornerhouse. Also it was all exceedingly cheap - £29 for the night including breakfast. As it was a damp and gloomy day, I was going to stay around for a while in the guest lounge watching TV, but on opening the door I was greeted by a large dog that was in there by itself and the Jeremy Kyle show was on the TV. Both are things I dislike! So I decided to go out and discover the delights of Carlisle.

I thought I might visit the castle and walked all the way round it trying to find the entrance. On asking someone, I discovered it was the Courthouse. The castle was the other end of the city! So I found my way to the Cathedral instead and the Tully Museum. This was very good and interesting but as with many museums there's too much to see in one visit. I then went to Wetherspoons and used their Wi-Fi to write and send my latest report to the Cleethorpes Chronicle.

I collected Ian from the station and we returned together to Wetherspoons for lunch. Ian is walking to Glasgow with me as we think it might be tricky. We enjoyed a restful day together and caught up with all our news.

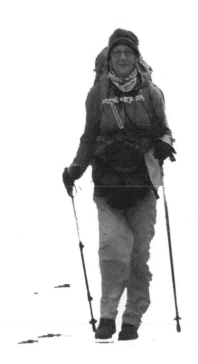

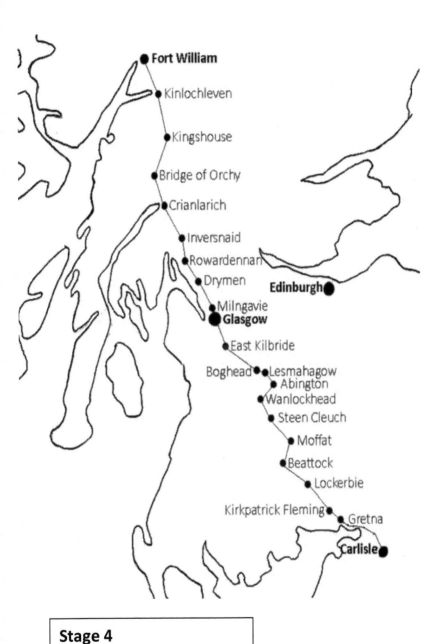

Fort William
Kinlochleven
Kingshouse
Bridge of Orchy
Crianlarich
Inversnaid
Rowardennan
Drymen
Edinburgh
Milngavie
Glasgow
East Kilbride
Boghead Lesmahagow
Abington
Wanlockhead
Steen Cleuch
Moffat
Beattock
Lockerbie
Kirkpatrick Fleming
Gretna
Carlisle

Stage 4

Carlisle to Fort William

Stage 4　　　　Carlisle to Fort William　24/6 – 11/7

	Ordinance Survey Map
Carlisle to Kirkpatrick Fleming (near Gretna) **Scotland** 18 miles	Explorer 315 & LR 85
Kirkpatrick Fleming to Lockerbie　13 miles	Landranger 85 & LR 78
Lockerbie to Beattock　17 miles	LR 78
Beattock to Moffat　3 miles	LR 78
Beattock to Steen Cleuch　12 miles	LR 78
Steen Cleuch to Wanlockhead　10 miles	LR 78
Wanlockhead/Abington/Lesmahagoe/ Boghead　13 m	LR 78 & LR 71
Boghead to East Kilbride　16 miles	LR 71 & LR 64
East Kilbride to Glasgow　10 miles	LR 64
Glasgow to Milngavie　9 miles	LR 64
Milngavie to Drymen　12 miles	LR 64
Drymen to Rowardennan YH　15 miles	Ex. 347
Rowardennan to Inversnaid Bunkhouse　8 miles	Ex. 364
Inversnaid Bunkhouse to Crianlarich YH　14 miles	Ex. 364
Crianlarich YH to Bridge of Orchy　14 miles	Ex. 364 & Ex. 377
Bridge of Orchy to Kingshouse　13 miles	Ex. 377
Kingshouse to Kinlochleven　9 miles	Ex. 384
Kinlochleven to Fort William　15 miles	Ex. 39
	Total　221 miles

18 walking days. Average 12.3 miles per day.　Days off: None

Saturday June 24th

Carlisle to Kirkpatrick Fleming (3 miles past Gretna)

Dumfries & Galloway, Scotland   *18 miles*

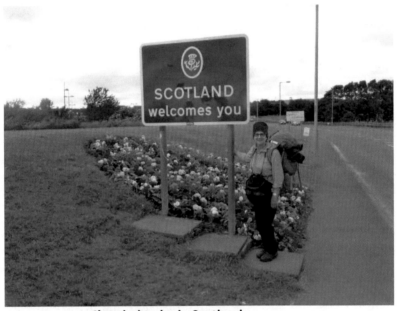

I'm glad to be in Scotland

It was a cool and windy day but sunny at times as Ian and I walked through the centre of Carlisle. We reached the outskirts and continued via roads and fields and by a river to the Gretna Outlet of shops where I got a refund at last for the pink poncho at Trespass. In Scotland at last! We celebrated in the café there with a chocolate éclair and a cup of tea.

We enjoyed going to Gretna Green and looking at the famous Blacksmith's shop, the scene of many runaway weddings. There was nobody around.

Then we walked along a long straight "B" road by a motorway. We reached the village of Kirkpatrick Fleming at 8pm and had a meal in the quiet old pub.

Our B & B was a ten minute walk from there. It was amazing! A beautiful old mansion where we were greeted by the charming lady who showed us to our delightful four-poster bedroom! We were invited to go down to the sumptuous lounge where we had tea and biscuits by the roaring fire and were joined by two other guests as well as the hostess. We had such a lovely evening chatting with them.

Sunday June 25th

Kirkpatrick Fleming to Lockerbie **Dumfries & Galloway** *13 miles*

Once again, it was another cool and windy day as we walked along some minor roads. We found a lovely hotel for lunch. We discovered a new Scottish border dessert – Ecclefechan tart. It's delicious. It is a pastry tart filled with caramel tasting dried fruit, walnuts and cherries.

Then we went on another "B" road next to a motorway for many miles. It was very noisy but easy, mostly flat walking. The verges were lovely with purple orchids, ragged robin, ox-eye daisies and foxgloves. The tall pink spikes of rosebay willow herb are just coming out too. We're now staying in a very pleasant place, the Crown Inn at Lockerbie and have just enjoyed the Sunday roast beef dinner followed by sticky toffee pudding. Delicious!

Monday June 26th

Lockerbie to Beattock   *Dumfries & Galloway*   *17 miles*

The Annandale Way

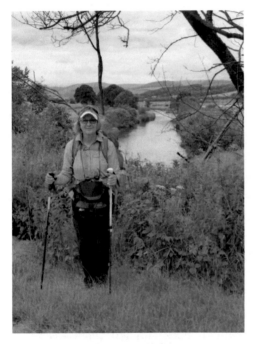

Ian and I went on the Annandale Way for a few miles which was a very pleasant path by the River Annan and through some woods and quiet lanes. The walking was easy and we could see the hills ahead. We had a lucky moment when we found a sealed pack of raspberries lying on the road! They were perfect, still in date too.

On the Annandale Way

The flowers we saw today were marsh valerian, meadow sweet, ragged robin and both tufted and bush vetch. The buttercup meadows are all cut for hay now. I'm so glad to be in Scotland as I love the hills and mountains, the wild heather moors and the lochs.

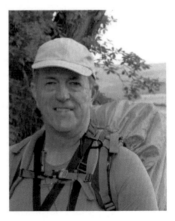

Ian

The walk today was very long but we played word games to pass the time and we sang too. We didn't get to the campsite until 7.15pm. It's in a lovely setting with hills quite close to us. However it's a bit midgy. So we're going to have our meal inside in the camp restaurant.

Tuesday June 27th

Beattock to Moffat   *Dumfries & Galloway*   *3 miles*

The Southern Upland Way

It rained all night and morning. We slept well in the tent despite the rain. However, it was tricky this morning with the rain as once you've crawled out there is no shelter. But we managed to have a good breakfast. Ian cooked his lovely porridge which we had with the raspberries that we found yesterday.

We walked on minor roads, the Southern Upland Way, and saw a deer and its baby racing across a field. The mother jumped the fence but the baby couldn't. I watched for ages. The fawn walked back and forth and so did its mother on the other side of the fence. Eventually the adult deer jumped back and led the baby to a different fence which she jumped. Again the baby couldn't do it. It was heart breaking. I didn't stay any longer as Ian had now gone ahead but I wonder what ensued. Farmers should think about leaving gaps for fawns to get through.

On arrival in the rain at Moffat, we went to a café for hot soup to warm us up. We were delighted to find Ecclefechan Tart again which we had with ice cream. Then we went to our B & B and had a relaxing afternoon followed by a pub meal in Moffat.

Wednesday June 28th

Beattock to Steen Cleuch   *Dumfries & Galloway*   *12 miles*

We caught the bus from Moffat back to Beattock and walked on the Southern Upland Way. This should be renamed the Southern Bogland Way as it is very boggy and today there were also very steep hills to go up and down. We climbed past coniferous forests and after six hours, we reached a high point where all around us

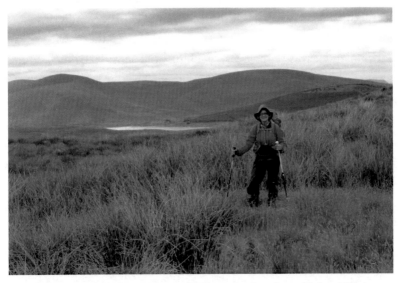

I'm exhausted after a steep climb on the Southern Upland Way

were wonderful mountain views and in the distance the Daer reservoir.

We had climbed up nearly 2000 feet. We then walked to the reservoir and made a wild camp there. Unfortunately, despite checking for midges before we decided to pitch the tent, as soon as the shelter and tent were up the midges came! We lit citronella incense sticks which helped a bit but we had to wear our midge nets over our heads so it was very difficult trying to eat the Bolognese and rice meal that Ian had cooked!

Thursday June 29th

Steen Cleuch up to hills 3 miles before Wanlockhead and back to road.

Dumfries & Galloway   *10 miles*

A very difficult day. Ian cooked breakfast on the roadside on the way. I was very down today. I really don't like camping. The rain didn't help. We walked on a good track to start with then climbed up Laight Hill. This is part of the Lowther Hills. The conditions were very bad. As well as it being steep and boggy there was a gale blowing and it was raining. On reaching Cold Moss Hill, it was so bad we were falling down with the gale blowing so hard and we weren't stable as we had our big packs on. We decided the conditions were too dangerous to continue as the mist was settling on the tops. We decided to turn towards where we could see a road in the distance and we climbed down. When we reached the road, we realised it was actually the same road that we'd started to climb up from, just a few hundred yards away! It had taken us many hours to do all that!

We thumbed a lift and the second vehicle stopped. It was a farmer in his smelly old van. He told us to throw our rucksacks in the back. I asked him where he wanted us to sit and he indicated the passenger seat. We had to clear the empty cans, newspapers and his scruffy hat and jacket off the seat before we could get in and I had to sit on Ian's knee. But we didn't care. We were saved! He took us to a warm café to recover. We tried to get a taxi but the only taxi driver in the town was on holiday we were told. When we tried the next town, we were told it was out of their area. I rang the Wanlockhead Inn where we were booked in for the night to stay in a wooden cabin called a pod. I asked if we could change that for a room inside as we were cold and soaked but were told they only had the pods outside. However, the kind owner came to fetch us.

The wooden pod was quite roomy and had a heater and a kettle. Nobody else was staying in the hotel. It's the highest pub in Scotland. It certainly would benefit from a woman's touch. It was not very clean and the food was basic but the guy let us dry our wet clothes in the tumble dryer and he was very pleasant. Also, he let us use his phone to book a B & B for tomorrow so we don't have to wild camp again. However the downside is that he doesn't stay on the premises at night so the toilet which is in the pub is only accessible from before midnight and opens again at 9.30am in the morning when he returns. So if we need the toilet in the night or early morning, it's the public toilet 300 yards down the road in the village!

Friday June 30th

Wanlockhead to Abington

Dumfries & Galloway & Lanarkshire   *10 miles*

Lesmahagow to Bogland   *3 miles*

We spent a reasonably good night in the pod. We were warm and managed to get all our things dry. We also managed OK with the toilet despite having to run to the public toilets 300 yards away in the village. But they were absolutely spotless! Better than the ones in the Wanlockhead Inn! We walked from the Inn along a "B" road which was undulating with nice views. We got to the service area at Abington where we caught a bus to Lesmahagow. This was because we didn't fancy another night wild camping again but could only find a B & B in a different area. However, this B & B is in a good area for the onward walk to Strathaven tomorrow. We had tea at the services, one mile past Abington.

From Lesmahagow, we walked three miles to our farm B & B at Bogland. It's actually a modern bungalow and is very nice. On the way, we were entertained by field voles darting in and out of their holes in the grassy verge. We saw at least twenty in the space of half an hour whereas in my whole life, I've only ever seen one in the wild.

Saturday July 1st

Dyke Croft Farm, Bogland to East Kilbride **Lanarkshire** *16 miles*

Ian and I walked from the farm in fine weather along a "B" road to Strathaven where our B & B is. We left our bags there. Then it started "mizzling" as we walked on minor roads to East Kilbride. We kept our spirits up by playing word games again. At East Kilbride, we ate at Wetherspoons then caught a bus back to Strathaven where we're staying. Our B & B, Rissons, is very posh with a restaurant. The owner was not particularly impressed when I told him about my walk. He said that a few years ago a man stayed with them who was doing Land's End to John O'Groats in bare feet! I can't think of anything worse! There are always stones, mud, gravel and hard roads. His feet must have been in a terrible state. The owner said that when he entered the house he put his shoes on.

Sunday July 2nd

East Kilbride to Glasgow   *10 miles*

We walked on some quiet minor roads from East Kilbride with some areas of countryside with farms and some pleasant villages with white houses. My back was aching today so Ian took some of my heavier things out of my rucksack to carry for me.

We had lunch in Asda then walked through the city until we reached our hotel, the Kelvingrove Park Hotel. We went to a local pub where we heard a jazz band and enjoyed a good meal.

Monday July 3rd

Glasgow to Milngavie **East Dunbartonshire** 9 miles

We decided to walk it backwards today so that Ian and I could stay in the same hotel for another night before he catches the train back. So we took the train to Milngavie and walked back along the Allander Water and a road back into Glasgow. It was a very pleasant and attractive walk along the river and through the Botanic Gardens and Kelvingrove Park. The weather was fine and sunny.

We had a relaxing afternoon watching Andy Murray win his first match of Wimbledon and also watched Heather Watson beat Jo Konta. It was great to catch some Wimbledon as I feared I wasn't going to be able to see any of it.

Ian left at 4pm to get the train back. He's been such a good help to me and I shall miss him. I booked an extra pick-up with Sherpa, the baggage company I'm using for four days of the West Highland Way, to take my rucksack tomorrow from Milngavie to Drymen. I prepared my maps and my rucksack and got my small day rucksack ready. What a relief it'll be to not have the great weight to carry!

Tuesday July 4th

Milngavie to Drymen **Stirlingshire** 12 miles

The West Highland Way

I'm looking forward to doing the West Highland Way even though I've done it before and remember what a tough walk it was. However, I was not very well when I did it last time so I want to enjoy it this time in full health. I remember how beautiful it was.

The West Highland Way, Scotland's first long distance footpath, was opened in 1980. It goes from Milngavie on the northern edge of

Glasgow to Fort William, at the foot of Ben Nevis. It uses ancient drove roads along which highlanders herded their cattle and sheep to market in the lowlands. It also uses military roads built by troops to help control the Jacobite clans. Old coaching roads and disused railway lines from the more recent past are also used for some of the route.

My first day was an easy introduction going along well-signed gravel paths through Mugdock Country Park, an area of beautiful deciduous woodlands and rushing streams. It then went onto a disused railway line. There were wild flower meadows to admire too: ragged robin, meadow sweet and valerian which is pale pink and not the same as the garden variety. There were some purple foxgloves, buttercups, small purple selfheal, and some giant hogweed. I also tasted my first wild raspberry of the year.

I chatted to about twenty walkers from America, France, Germany, Holland and Sweden who all started about the same time as I did from Milngavie. Eventually, we arrived at the village of Drymen. I'm staying at the Hawthorns B & B where I stayed before with my friends. It's been taken over by another couple and it's much improved now and the new owners are very pleasant and friendly. My room is perfect with a TV and a radiator that came on. (They don't always as it's the summer, but you often need some warmth at night, especially if you've got clothes to dry.) There are also some nice biscuits in the room, again this doesn't always happen. B & B's seem to be cutting back.

In the evening, I joined my new walking friends at the Clachan pub for a meal and we enjoyed chatting. I also managed to watch some more Wimbledon though both Djokovic and also Federer's opponents pulled out of their matches through injury so I only saw two half matches. Very disappointing!

Wednesday July 5th

Drymen to Rowardennan YH   ***Stirlingshire***   *15 miles*

It was a fine, sunny day as I set off alone to walk along forest tracks and on minor roads with superb views of Loch Lomond and the mountains. There were flowers to admire along the way: pink valerian, yellow St John's-wort, rosebay willowherb, bird's-foot-trefoil and the tiny yellow tormentil. I caught up with the others that I met yesterday and we were joined by about 100 German students climbing Conic Hill. I remember it being a tough climb from last time when I did it but this time it was easy. So it should be after 830 miles of walking up and down hills! It's a steady climb at first then a bit of a scramble to take you up to the first rocky peak. After that, there are a couple of small hilltops to cross to take you to the viewpoint over Loch Lomond. We took photos of the views and each other. There were lots of steps and rocky paths to climb down, then a forest path. This led to Balmaha where there were cafés and a visitor centre. I had some cake and a cup of tea and sat with Alex, the French young lady and her 16-year-old son and her friend. I really like them.

I had a leisurely walk alone back along the shore of Loch Lomond. It was so beautiful! Then I suddenly realised I'd still got seven more miles to go and it was 4.30pm already. So I decided to go on the road and did some fast walking to Rowardennan Hotel. I enjoyed Cullen skink, a creamy potato and leek soup with warm bread. The TV was on in the bar and so I watched Nadal play some tennis before I set off to the Youth Hostel. It's very crowded in the dormitory and as usual, I'm left with a top bunk. Unfortunately, the girl in the top bunk next to me has a streaming cold. I'm hoping I don't catch it.

Thursday July 6th

Rowardennan YH to Inversnaid Bunkhouse **Stirlingshire**   *8 miles*

It was a fine but damp day as I walked alone through the woods above Loch Lomond. The path was rocky at times with some tricky crossings of stream inlets and also boulders to climb over. It was very up-and-down but I managed it fine. The midges were out, being damp and still; perfect conditions for them! It was OK if you didn't stop. I stopped briefly by the loch for my lunch. Big mistake! I had to put my midge net on and had to keep walking up and down.

I've found out what the yellow flower is that's growing all over the woods. It's wood cow-wheat. It has pairs of flowers growing each side of the stem. It's about six inches high.

Eventually, I reached the Inversnaid Hotel where I enjoyed two pieces of delicious lemon drizzle cake and a pot of tea. Then I had to walk half a mile uphill to the Inversnaid Bunkhouse where I'm in a private room with two single beds in it. It's very small and has no sink and no TV. There's no TV anywhere in the building. This is most disappointing as I was hoping to watch some Wimbledon.

I had haggis, neeps and tatties tonight in the restaurant upstairs. It was OK but not as good as I'd hoped. You have to have it when in Scotland. I did have the vegetarian one as I don't like the idea of the disgusting things that go into the meat version.

Friday July 7th

Inversnaid Bunkhouse to Crianlarich YH **Perthshire** *14 miles*

The first five miles from Inversnaid were tough. The terrain was the hardest I've encountered on my journey. There were steep rocky paths with huge boulders to climb and many streams to cross, jumping from rock to rock. Of course, there was no one to help me. If Ian had been with me he'd have given me a hand. I have to be determined and I know I can do these things now. I have to.

Just when I was exhausted, I saw the sign for Rob Roy's cave. Last time I was here, I decided not to visit it due to being too tired but I thought I'd better go this time as I'd probably not return here. It was another precipitous scramble down huge rocks to the loch shore. The cave was more of a cleft in a massive boulder but it was enough to spark the images of Rob Roy planning who to kidnap and imprison next.

The loch side path goes along Loch Lomond passing through much natural oak woodland. Eventually, it left the loch side and the woodland. It opened out. There were more flowers here: the delicate, tiny white eyebright, the pale purple fragranced wild thyme, the pretty purple selfheal and yellow St John's-wort.

At Invernarnan, the loch came to an end and the West Highland Way continued by the River Falloch with several impressive waterfalls. On the bottom step of a wooden bridge, a beautifully patterned common lizard was resting. At Beinglas Farm, I went to a bar and saw the French people. Alex has to stop the walk due to knee pain and she told me that yesterday she had to catch the boat to this place. There are no roads nearby if you have an injury. It's all down to boats. They're camping near here. Hugo, her son, and Jasmine, her friend, walked today but all are having to go home tomorrow. Quel dommage!

The day was long but there were lovely views and I saw a lot of people but none I'd seen before today. I think some will definitely have given up. If you're not fit, it's a very tough walk.

I'm now at the Youth hostel and I am actually in a bottom bunk for a change! There are only two German girls here at the moment. There was no food available in the Hostel so I had to walk to the pub in the village – not far. What a treat it was! I caught Andy Murray's match. It was fantastic! Everyone in the pub was silent and enthralled. I had a glass of wine and a venison burger for only £8!

Saturday July 8th

Crianlarich to Bridge of Orchy   **Perthshire & Argyll**   *14 miles*

I was disappointed to find that there was only a continental breakfast available at the Youth Hostel this morning. And even more so to find you have to wash up here! However, there was a fantastic drying room and a good shower. Everywhere was spotlessly clean. I enjoyed chatting to an older lady over breakfast.

It was a fine sunny day as I set off to walk uphill through the forest to reach the West Highland Way. I continued to climb uphill along the River Fillon past the ruined Augustinian Priory of St Fillan. Fillan came from Ireland in the 13th Century to spread Christianity to the Scots and the Picts in this area. The priory was built after his death in recognition of his teachings and later, he became a saint. The old burial ground nearby contained, among other graves, four early medieval cross slabs dating from around the seventh or eighth century. They are very rare and are covered with turf to protect them so I didn't see them.

I reached a café at Strathfillan Wigwams Campsite for coffee and a banana. An unexpected delight!

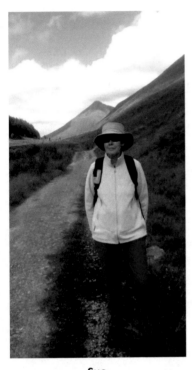

Sue

At Tyndrum, I met my old school friend Sue who now lives on the Isle of Bute which is not that far from here. We had a wonderful afternoon chatting. It's always great to see her and we pick up seamlessly from when we last saw each other which was about three years ago I think.

It was easy walking on good paths, some uphill, with wonderful mountain views all round. Sue is not a walker but she managed seven miles before being picked up by Pete, her husband, at Bridge of Orchy.

Sue and Pete went home after they had taken me back to Tyndrum in their car where Patsy was waiting in the camper van. We had a nice evening drinking, eating and chatting. However, the van is rather a long way from the toilet block.

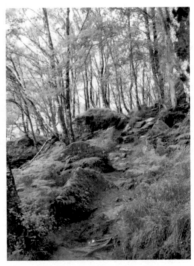

The West Highland Way

Sunday July 9th

Bridge of Orchy to Kingshouse   **Argyll**   *13 miles*

It was rainy all day. And it was also very midgy as the little creatures like damp weather. Patsy walked two miles with me over the grassy moors to the Inveroran Hotel where we enjoyed coffee and fruit cake. There were lots of walkers today. I walked up and over Rannoch Moor. Despite the poor weather, I loved it. The mountains were bathed in mist and clouds hung between them giving them an ethereal splendour.

I kept walking because of the threat of midges and only stopped once high up on the heather moors for lunch. A group of Scottish walkers passed by wearing some greenery in their hats and round their necks. I asked them about it and they said it was bog myrtle which keeps the midges off. It was growing by the side of the path in many places so I picked some and stuck it in my hat. It certainly helped!

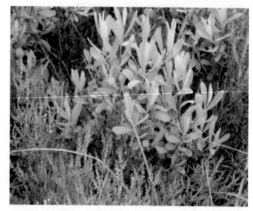

On arrival at Kingshouse, the white old inn nestling under the high mountains, I discovered it was closed for refurbishment. I have stayed here before and it

Bog myrtle deters the midges

was a lovely place. However, they have put up a new wooden temporary building with no character but I enjoyed a cup of tea and some Scottish shortbread there. Patsy met me. We took photos near the wild deer, including one with big antlers. People feed them; that's why they come down from the mountains.

Midges have got in the camper van tonight! Both of us have bites on our arms and my arms were covered up! We dried our wet clothes on a washing line we've set up in the van.

Monday July 10th

Kingshouse to Kinlochleven   **Argyll**   *9 miles*

I walked alone from Kingshouse dreading the next big climb, the Devil's Staircase. I remember how hard it was from the last time I did it. It took forty minutes to climb up and it wasn't too bad at all. There were fabulous views as I was going up.

Two hundred yards from the top, there was a very exciting handwritten sign – "shop at top". I kept visualising a cup of steaming frothy coffee. Unfortunately, when I reached the top, it was an unmanned small tent with fizzy drinks for a pound and an honesty box. I applaud the business acumen of some undoubtedly young person but it was very disappointing for me. I don't even like fizzy drinks. However, the tremendous mountain views all around were worth the climb, despite the light rain that started. There were quite a lot of other walkers on this stretch who were very friendly.

I saw the starry yellow flowers again that I had thought were St John's-wort. I've discovered they are actually bog asphodel. It can grow at high altitudes and is especially happy on boggy moors. Patsy has a very good flower book in the camper van.

I walked to Kinlochleven which is in a spectacular setting surrounded by imposing mountains. It's a centre for outdoor tourism and mountain sports. The Ice Factor is a popular place. It has, among other things, the biggest indoor ice climbing facility and the UK's largest rock climbing wall. Patsy met me and we went to a pub and watched Wimbledon. Murray won again. Hooray!

Tuesday July 11th

Kinlochleven to Fort William **Inverness-shire** *15 miles*

This was a wonderful last day of the West Highland Way. The sun was shining. I climbed up through woodland at first, for forty minutes. Then I was on an undulating wide path through the mountains. This had been an old military road. The scenery was absolutely stunning; rushing rivers, tumultuous waterfalls and mountains in every direction. The path was stony with many streams to cross. I saw a lovely flower that is new to me – yellow mountain saxifrage growing on rocky wet ground.

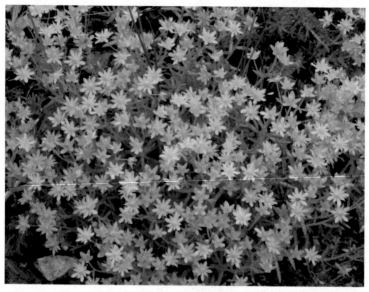

Mountain saxifrage

As I was resting on a felled tree stump, an older man (Rob) stopped to chat. I found out that he is doing Land's End to John O'Groats too! We had a long chat and compared our routes. His wife is supporting him by being the back-up driver. He gave me £5 for my charity.

120

Eventually, the massive bulk of Ben Nevis was next to me. A rain shower started and as I walked by the mountain there was a beautiful rainbow low over it. It seemed like a fitting end to a glorious walk.

As I was walking into the town, a Spanish guy approached me. He said he was thinking of climbing Ben Nevis tomorrow and would I recommend it? I think he thought I looked such a wreck I must have just climbed it. I told him that I'd never climbed it but I'd seen people going up it early in the morning so I knew it would take many hours. He wanted to know if it was risky. I suggested he ask someone who had actually climbed it. However, he told me he'd walked the Camino in Spain so I'm sure he'd be fit enough.

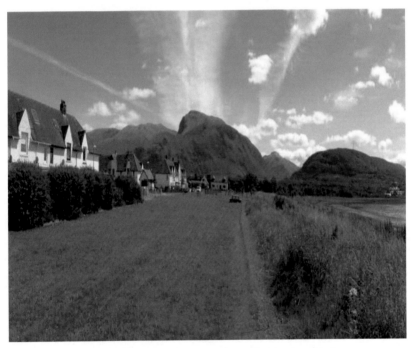

Fort William with Ben Nevis in the background

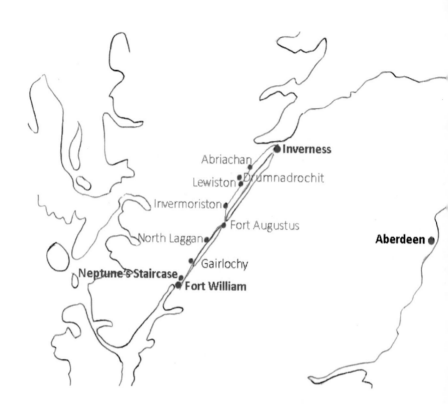

Stage 5

Fort William to Inverness

Stage 5   Fort William to Inverness   12/7 – 19/7

	Ordinance Survey Map	
Fort William to Neptune's Staircase	4 miles	Ex. 392
Neptune's Staircase to Gairlochy	8 miles	Ex. 392 & Ex. 400
Gairlochy to North Laggan	14 miles	Ex. 400
North Laggan to Fort Augustus	10 miles	Ex. 400
Fort Augustus to Invermoriston	9 miles	Ex. 400 & & Ex. 416
Invermoriston to Lewiston	15 miles	Ex. 416
Lewiston to Abriachan	9 miles	Ex. 416
Abriachan to Inverness	13 miles	Ex. 416

Total   82 miles.   8 walking days.   Average 10.2 miles per day. Days off: 0

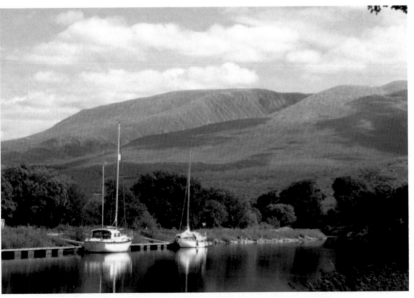

Along the Caledonian Canal with Ben Nevis in the background

Wednesday July 12th

Fort William to Neptune's Staircase 4 miles

The Great Glen Way

This was really a day off but I thought I might as well walk a bit so Patsy and I walked in warm sunshine together for a mile and a half to a café in a distillery.

It's unfortunate (or maybe not) that I'm passing all these distilleries as I don't even like whisky! When Patsy left to go back to the camper van, I walked a quarter of a mile in the wrong direction as it was rather confusing. We were on a diversion from the Great Glen Way because of some work going on along the footpath. I found the right way and had a lovely walk by the loch then the Caledonian Canal under the shadow of Ben Nevis. It was looking splendid in the sun. I might climb it next year as a tribute to being seventy! I was thinking of the Spanish guy I saw yesterday and wondered if he was climbing it. It was perfect weather today for it.

The Great Glen Way is a 79 mile trail from Fort William to Inverness following sections of Thomas Telford's historic Caledonian Canal along the towpaths. It also goes up onto the forest roads and tracks and along lochs including Loch Ness. I met Patsy by Neptune's Staircase. This is a series of eight locks lifting boats twenty metres. It takes ninety minutes to climb the staircase in a boat. I did it in five. One of the few occasions when walking is the quickest way to go!

We drove to the same hotel as yesterday to watch the tennis on the TV there. Unfortunately we saw Murray get beaten by a Canadian due to injury. But at least he didn't retire injured like some have done this Wimbledon.

We went to our new campsite which is right under Ben Nevis. A fantastic location! We sat outside in the sun for a change as there were very few midges. We have to change tomorrow's campsite as we'd booked one at Gairloch and we've found out that it's miles and miles away from Gairlochy where we need to be!

Thursday July 13th

Neptune's Staircase to Gairlochy   **Inverness-shire**   *8 miles*

I had an easy walk along the canal. The flowers along the bank were lady's bedstraw, harebells (the Scottish bluebell), clover, tufted vetch and valerian. There was hardly anyone about, just a few cyclists. I walked fast as I wanted to get back for the tennis to see the Wimbledon semi-final – Venus Williams and Jo Conta. Patsy and I watched it in a pub. Unfortunately, Venus won but it was an enjoyable match to watch. We're in a new campsite tonight near Gairlochy.

Friday July 14th

Gairlochy to North Laggan   **Inverness-shire**   *14 miles*

I started at Gairlochy Swing Bridge and had a long woodland walk in showery weather on forest roads. Walking all day I only saw two German girls and one man. There were a few cyclists. Patsy joined me for short stretches from time to time. There were not many views because of the trees. It was by Loch Lochy. This was an area used for sea-faring training for commandos in the Second World War. They used live ammunition in their mock battles as they were trained to shoot to miss. Sounds very scary to me! It was quite difficult to find toilet stops due to a steep bank on one side going down to the loch and a steep upward incline on the other side with a stream.

I saw two water voles scurrying across the path. It's always a delight to see something like that. They are one of my favourite creatures. In the woods, I saw wood vetch again that Linda and I had seen on the Dales Way. It is a beautiful white and mauve trailing plant. The yellow cow-wheat flower was also growing in the woods. I eventually reached the end of Loch Lochy at Laggan. After that, there was a mile stretch along the Caledonian Canal while I was still in the forest. I met Patsy at North Laggan car park.

Saturday July 15th

North Laggan to Fort Augustus   **Inverness-shire**   *10 miles*

The forest road by Loch Lochy and Loch Oich uses one of General Wade's military roads. They were built to allow troops to control rebellious Highlanders. The forest road was very long and straight and when the commandos had to first march down it, they were accompanied by a rousing pipe band to raise their spirits. In the continual rain that I had today, I could have done with that band to cheer me on but at least I had a parade of tall foxgloves each side of me to encourage my marching.

A long stretch of the Caledonian Canal followed with flowers on the bank including white ox-eye daisies, yellow St John's-wort and the creamy, fragrant, blowzy meadowsweet.

At last, I reached Fort Augustus which is a charming village with pubs, cafes and interesting shops as well as boats along the canal to look at. You can go on a boat trip on Loch Ness to look for the monster if you have the time! Which we don't!

There were a few more walkers and cyclists today, probably because it's Saturday. Patsy and I found a café that put the TV on especially for us so we were able to watch the Wimbledon Final. It was excellent. Muguruza from Spain beat Venus Williams. Hooray!

I sorted my rucksack out and left a few more things with Patsy as I now have to carry my bag all the way to John O'Groats. Patsy leaves tomorrow.

Sunday July 16th

Fort Augustus to Invermoriston   **Inverness-shire**   *9 miles*

Patsy walked with me a short way then I said goodbye to her. I'm very grateful to her for all the help she's given me. My bag is now 22 lbs in weight as I have left out as much as possible but it still felt heavy.

The forest tracks were undulating by Loch Ness. I only saw the loch for about ten minutes though because of the trees masking the view. It is possible to get better views if you take a higher track but I wasn't prepared to do that because of the heavy rucksack.

I rang the B & B and discovered it was not at Altsigh as I had thought but at Invermoriston which was so much nearer. It meant I had every chance of getting there in time to watch the Wimbledon men's final! And I did! Federer beat Cilic. However, it was not a very exciting match. But it meant that Federer won his eighth Wimbledon title which is a record. He's the first person to do that.

It was a lovely evening. I walked a hundred yards down the road to the pub and was invited to join a pleasant young couple, Vanessa and Paul, at their table. I had a delicious summer pudding. On returning to the B & B I had an extra treat – I watched Poldark from my bed. Wonderful!

Monday July 17th

Invermoriston to Lewiston (near Drumnadrochit)

Inverness-shire   *15 miles*

It was another long day walking in the forest and quite hilly. Carrying my bag was tiring. There were a few fleeting views of Loch Ness but it was a more interesting path than yesterday. And the sun was shining.

I had an interesting time at an unexpected café that was attached to a pottery in the forest. I sat outside and an eccentric old man came to chat to me. He had long white hair and was wearing a sun hat, shorts and sandals. His chest was bare. He was carrying a long hand-made walking stick. He told me he lived in the big house next to the pottery. He was from Devon. On telling him about my walk, he said he knew of a good way to get to John O'Groats. He went to his house and fetched a road map. He suggested a route that went on a "B" road north from Drumnadrochit and then along the coast east to John O'Groats. I could tell it would add miles to my walk but humoured him and said it was certainly worth considering.

The café and pottery owner, on learning of my charity walk, let me have the tea and cake for free. So I kept the £4.50 as a donation. I walked happily down the road to Lewiston picking ripe bilberries to eat as I went towards my B & B. High in the sky, I saw a red kite soaring. The B & B that I'm staying at is Glen Rowan where I stayed before. However, it has changed hands and unfortunately it's not got the same wonderful ambience as before although the new lady owner is very nice. It was owned by a lovely couple who would give us a lift to and from the next place so we could easily stay two nights here. The jolly proprietor used to serve breakfast wearing a kilt and Scottish music would be playing.

Tuesday July 18th

Lewiston to Abriachan　　　　　**Inverness-shire**　　　*9 miles*

It was a warm and sunny day today as I set off to continue the Great Glen Way. It was more interesting today with the forest opening out to reveal more views of Loch Ness including the mighty ruins of medieval Urquhart Castle. Throughout the Middle Ages, Urquhart Castle was the centre of a vast productive estate. The laird of Urquhart controlled the fertile pastures near Loch Ness and the rich hunting grounds in the mountains nearby.

The weather was lovely and it brought out more walkers and cyclists. However, there were more hills today. The paths were always stony and narrow in parts. There was lots of heather around.

I arrived at the edge of the forest at Abriachan to meet the taxi to take me back to the B & B. However, it was too early, so on seeing an interesting hand-painted sign with my favourite word on - Café - I made my way towards it. It was a narrow path with bushes on either side. There were various roughly painted signs encouraging you to keep going e.g. hot drinks, cake, eco café. It turned out to be at least half a mile away. It made me wonder how far would I go for a cup of tea? The good thing was that I didn't have to carry my big bag as I'm spending two nights at the B & B that I was in yesterday and using a taxi to return there today and to go back to today's finishing point tomorrow. This is because there is no accommodation in Abriachan.

When I eventually arrived at the eco café, it was deserted except for a few chickens. It was a ramshackle place. There was a bell hung on a rope which I duly rang and a flamboyant, smiling woman emerged to see what I wanted. There was no list of food up anywhere but I asked for a cup of tea and some cake. It seemed there was only one type of cake and she brought it and left the bill asking me to leave the money on the table when I'd finished. She also had a chat with me and I told her about my walk. She took my photo for her Facebook page.

I must admit the cake was very nice but I nearly fainted when I saw the bill - £11. It was £3 for the tea and £8 for the cake! I didn't know whether to leave what I thought it was worth on the table or confront her. I decided on the latter. I rang the bell again and she duly appeared, still smiling. I told her I thought there'd been a mistake on the bill. She replied that there was no mistake. I told her it was much too expensive and that yesterday I'd had the same at another café for £4.50. She insisted that the price was correct and it was all home-made. I offered to pay her £6 (which was still too much) and that was all. She kept on and on about how expensive it was to live out here and I told her that my charity walk was costing me a lot of money too. In the end I'm sorry to say I got fed up with it and just gave her the £11. But it did spoil my day.

However, when I left, I managed to etch out with a stone on her wooden café sign "cake £8". And tonight I went on her Facebook page. There I was, smiling with my piece of cake! I wrote on her comments page about the extortionate prices. And I got my friends to also put on some comments like "shocking!" and "the highest prices in the highest café in Scotland!" I feel a bit better now.

On the short walk to the pub this evening I heard the evocative sound of bagpipes playing. It sounded like they were being played in a meadow a long way away. On speaking to a local I found out it was Duncan practising in the fields. I think that's the perfect way to hear bagpipes – for no more than ten minutes and far away! I managed to have another Scottish delicacy at the pub tonight – cranachan; that's raspberries with cream flavoured with honey, whisky and oatmeal. Delicious!

Abriachan to Inverness   **Inverness-shire**   *13 miles*

At breakfast this morning, I met a man of 81 years old who is cycling to John O'Groats from Land's End with his wife as back up in the car. They've ridden tandems together all over the world before this. He told me he'd had a check-up with his doctor to see if it would harm him to do this challenge and was told that no pill in the world is as good as exercise. He was looking and feeling fit and happy. Funnily enough he's actually cycling north from Drumnadrochit on the route described by the old man I met in the café two days ago! I'm sure it's a very pretty way to go but it must be more miles than my intended route.

It was warm and sunny as I walked alone along the last easy part of the Great Glen Way to Inverness. I'd been dropped off by a taxi at the point where I finished yesterday although I had to repeat the walk along the trail past the infamous and expensive eco-café of yesterday as the taxi dropped me off at the nearest road.

However, as I walked along the path, with open country views of mountains and farmland, I met about a dozen walkers going the other way. I stopped each one and warned them about the extortionate price of cake in the eco-café that they'd be passing. They were grateful for the tip. I passed through some pleasant woodland and eventually, the path climbed up next to a small reservoir with wonderful views of the city of Inverness below. The path gradually wound its way down and the last part was a walk along the Caledonian Canal again and then a lovely park with a river and the canal accompanying me into the city. I walked past the Cathedral and the Castle. I continued through the city, trying to find the Youth Hostel.

I met an old man who was also looking for the Youth Hostel. We walked along together, chatting, and when I told him about my walk he was very impressed and shook my hand. He said how much he respected me for my achievement and that meeting me had made his day! It certainly improved mine too!

I met Sue who's going to walk with me for three days. She came up here on the train, with her bike. Sue is an old walking friend of mine from Cleethorpes. In 2007, we did The Coast to Coast together, our first long distance walk. Sue now does lots of cycling and after walking with me she's going to do a long cycle ride in Scotland. We discovered there were no evening meals served in the Youth Hostel, despite it being a huge modern place. So we went out to Morrisons for some food to bring back in to eat. We had a good evening chatting.

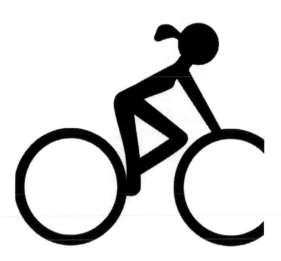

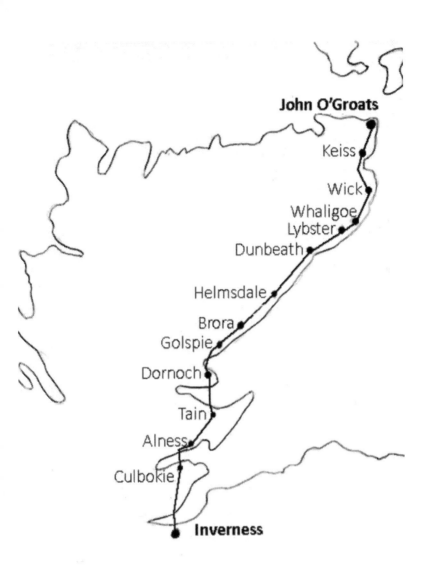

John O'Groats

Keiss

Wick

Whaligoe
Lybster

Dunbeath

Helmsdale

Brora

Golspie

Dornoch

Tain

Alness

Culbokie

Inverness

Stage 6

Inverness to John O'Groats

Stage 6   **Inverness to John O'Groats**   **20/7/17 – 1/8/17**

		Ordinance Survey Map
Inverness to Culbokie	13 ½ miles	Explorer 416
Culbokie to Alness	9 miles	Landranger 21
Alness to Tain	13 ½ miles	LR 21
Tain to Dornoch	10 miles	LR 21
Dornoch to Golspie	14 miles	LR 17
Golspie to Brora	8 miles	LR 17
Brora to Helmsdale	15 miles	LR 17
Helmsdale to Dunbeath	15 miles	LR 17
Dunbeath to Lybster	10 miles	LR 12
Lybster to Whaligoe	6 miles	LR 12
Whaligoe to Wick	10 ½ miles	LR 12
Wick to Keiss	12 ½ miles	LR 12
Keiss to John O'Groats	12 miles	LR 12

**Total   149 miles   13 walking days.   Average 11.6 miles per day.
Days off: None**

**Total mileage 1194 miles from Land's End to John O'Groats on
footpaths, fields and roads.**

Thursday July 20th

Inverness to Culbokie   **Inverness-shire**   *13 ½ miles*

Sue and I had a lovely easy walk from Inverness Youth Hostel passing the imposing Inverness Castle. It was "mizzling" and there was light rain through the morning. We went through the shopping area and crossed a suspension bridge, Kessock Bridge, across the Moray Firth. It was very noisy with the traffic and not very pleasant although the views were good. We were approaching the Black Isle area. I've never been north of Inverness before. Once we got over the bridge, it was rather pleasant walking on quiet minor roads that went by farm land with cows and sheep. There were little hamlets with attractive white cottages and in the distance the mountains of the Western Highlands. The weather improved and was dry and cloudy with no wind.

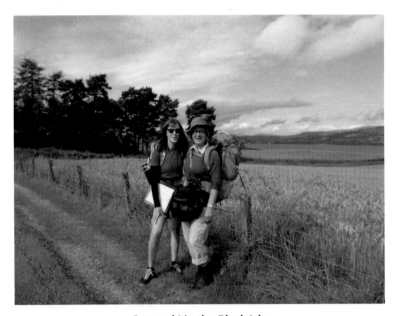

Sue and I in the Black Isle

On reaching the village of Culbokie, we found the pub, a friendly place, and had apple and walnut salad with chips. We had a lovely chocolate flake ice cream from the local shop too. After another half mile, we reached our wonderful B & B, Netherton Farm. It's an old building with lovely old furniture. The ladies who run it are warm and friendly. They welcomed us with a cup of tea, something that sadly is not usually the case these days. There are fantastic views over the Cromarty Firth and the mountains beyond are wreathed in clouds. It's very still and calm. A peaceful place. The pièce de résistance was being able to luxuriate in a deep bath. A perfect end to a lovely day.

Friday July 21st

Culbokie to Alness   ***Ross-shire***   *9 miles*

It was a fine day today as Sue and I walked through pleasant pastoral countryside. We crossed the Cromarty Bridge over the Cromarty Firth. It was not as noisy as the previous bridge but still very long. It was a lovely walk with lots of rosebay willowherb at the sides of the roads and also wild raspberries; some were very big and juicy!

At lunchtime, we found a pub and had a latte coffee. We arrived at the Commercial Hotel at Alness to discover that I'd actually booked the Commercial Hotel at Wishart, Motherwell by mistake on Booking.com! Protracted pleading with Booking.com did no good at all and I have to pay £50 to cancel it as I haven't given the required notice. (The room was £100). Fortunately, there was a twin room available here for £75. We went to the Co-op and got a small bottle of wine each and I got a can of Baileys and a bar of chocolate too to make me feel a bit better. This was after we'd had a fish and chips supper in the local fish shop. We then watched TV.

Saturday July 22nd

Alness to Tain   **Ross-shire**   *13 ½ miles*

It was easy walking again today in fine weather as Sue and I walked on mainly flat, minor roads. There were fields with cows on either side of the road. How wonderful to not have to go through those fields! There were some cottages too. We talked and laughed all the way.

Tain is quite a big village and a Royal burgh. It's got a few imposing buildings and shops with pretty hanging baskets. Ian arrived unexpectedly tonight at our B & B. We weren't expecting him till tomorrow. We all went out to eat at a lovely restaurant at the station.

Sunday July 23rd

Tain to Dornoch   **Sutherland**   *10 miles*

Sue left today to go back on the train to Inverness where she'll collect her bike from the Youth Hostel and do a long cycle ride before returning home to Cleethorpes. Ian will now be with me to John O'Groats. Most people walk on the A9 and the A99 in this area to get to John O'Groats. We decided it would be too dangerous so we've downloaded the information from the internet to go on a new route. This has been devised by an American, Jay Wilson, who lives up here in Helmsdale. It's a route that goes between the A9 and A99 and the sea. When the minor roads run out, we'll try it.

It was easy flat walking today. After some drizzle first thing, the weather was fine. Ian and I crossed the Dornoch Firth by a long bridge on the A9 then minor roads to Dornoch. Dornoch is a lovely small town with a cathedral! There are castle walls, imposing buildings and attractive flowers everywhere. We are in a spectacular looking hotel just by the sea and a golf course. However, it is quite

137

run down and needs refurbishment. When we got to our room, we found the previous guests' towels still in the bathroom! We threw them onto a huge pile of dirty linen that was outside our room. The TV is old fashioned but at least it works. The bathroom is small and outdated. Ian and I had a relaxing afternoon and went to a nice restaurant in a pub in the town. Then we watched Poldark.

Monday July 24th

Dornoch to Golspie   **Sutherland**   *14 miles*

The trouble with walking round this area is that there are so many lochs and firths to get round. Today it was sunny and warm. We walked on minor roads and footpaths. We had to get round a large stretch of water, Loch Fleet. It took us all day to do this. If there'd been a ferry it would have been much quicker! We tried to avoid the A9 as much as possible so we walked close to the water through long grass, rocks and pools. There were patches of pretty, purple sea asters and pink ragged robin flowers. Eventually, we had to climb up the bank to return to the main road as we needed to cross a bridge. However, there was no easy way to get through the prickly gorse on the steep bank. Luckily, Ian found a plank and tunnelled his way through the gorse so that we could climb up on to the A9. It was not too awful but bad enough.

When I was at the infamous eco-café, the stingy woman there told me about a lady hiker who was walking from John O'Groats to Land's End. She was walking on the A9 when her backpack was clipped by a lorry and she was thrown into the ditch. She was saved by a passing postman. She arrived at the café bloody and bruised. So that's one reason why we felt we shouldn't walk on the main roads.

We crossed the bridge on the A9 and then went on a forest path that is mentioned in Jay Wilson's alternative route. We went through a field of cows, calves and a massive bull with a ring in its nose but they ignored us! However, I was very nervous going by them. Ian didn't even notice the bull as it was sitting down! When we got through the field, they all came to the gate to peer at us. This is one reason why I like having Ian with me. It makes me feel more confident in scary situations.

We walked through a barley field and down a lane. We came to a lovely forest and saw our first proper sign for the John O'Groats Trail although we had seen some splashes of white paint on gates and walls. Jay Wilson has a band of volunteers who are helping him make this route. They are putting in stiles so you don't have to climb walls and fences and they're building bridges so you don't have to wade through rivers. However, it's not yet finished and we know that we will have to do some climbing of walls and fording of rivers. It's supposed to be going to be finished in two years' time. They have to get permission from the various land owners to carry out these changes.

We eventually arrived at our comfortable B & B, The Granite Guest House, at 7.15pm. We had fish and chips in a restaurant. It was very welcome!

Tuesday July 25th

Golspie to Brora   **Sutherland**   *8 miles*

Today I felt like I was on holiday! We had a lovely day in fine weather walking along beach paths and on the sand and pebbles. We passed Dunrobin fairy-tale castle. We decided to visit it but when we got to the entrance we changed our mind. It was heaving with tourists and coach loads more just arriving. So I just had a photo with the piper at the door.

Ian and I passed a well-preserved broch, Carn Liath, an Iron Age Pictish home. Brochs are the tallest prehistoric buildings in Britain. They are 2000 year old stone fortified houses for chieftains and at least 700 brochs once existed across northern and western Scotland. Now there are the ruins of about 200 left. They had two concentric dry stone walls and huge windowless towers. Ian went to visit this ruined one and went in various small underground rooms. I wished I'd gone too when he told me about it.

Along the pebbly beach we saw seals, oyster catchers, herons and cormorants. There were some lovely flowers on the beach: tall yellow sow thistles, golden ragwort, sea mayweed and sea rocket.

At one point we went up the cliff to a "mezzanine" level half way up, and discovered a hidden valley. There were delightful butterflies and flowers there. It was lovely and warm. We came down a steep cliffside path to a beautiful glade with a high waterfall, Sputie burn. There was a rocky pool surrounded by wild flowers. Climbing up the cliffs were the flowers of lady's mantle.

We eventually reached the village of Brora. There's one main street (the A9 goes through the village) and some shops and a café. We're staying at the Sutherland Inn. We enjoyed a good meal in the pub tonight.

Wednesday July 26th

Brora to Helmsdale   **Sutherland**   *15 miles*

Today was a very hard day. We were walking for eleven hours. It started off OK walking by the golf course and it was lovely on the sandy and pebbly beach. We saw oystercatchers and ringed plovers. Black backed gulls and Arctic terns were doing aerobatics in the sky and seals and eider ducks were swimming in the rough sea to entertain us. However, when we followed the route inland it became more challenging. We climbed up from the beach and there was no path; we were walking through long tufts of grass. This deteriorated to high bracken ending in a river which we had to cross. We had come prepared. We put on our plastic bags over our boots and secured them with rubber bands. The river was under a railway bridge with a rocky cliff on one side. Strangely, there was a ladder propped up under the bridge. We did think about laying it across the river to get across but then one of us would have had to take it back again so we decided it wasn't a good idea. There was a rocky weir going across so it was very scary trying to cross. I was worried I might slip and fall into the deep rushing water by the weir. But luckily I didn't.

After that adventure, we climbed up the rocky cliff side and continued through high bracken, nettles and undergrowth. This led to the beach where we had to cross a wide river outlet. It looked as if you could easily paddle across it. However, there was a deeper creek within it and Ian noticed it. He called out to me to jump across it. Of course my legs are not as long as Ian's. I fell in onto my knees so the rest of the walk I had to contend with soaking feet and legs.

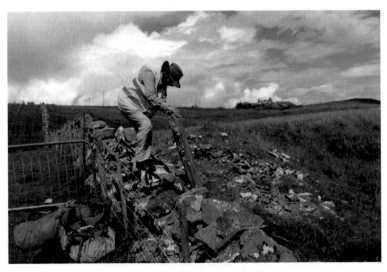

I'm struggling over a wall

We were trying to follow Jay Wilson's directions. Some of them weren't right and we wandered round one field for ages trying to find which fence or wall to cross to get across the burn. We eventually decided on a fence to cross. We used our foam pipe insulator over the barbed wire but there was an unexpectedly deep landing!

We fought through more high bracken and nettles and crossed the burn. However, immediately there was another challenge. It was an almost vertical bank which we climbed or rather, crawled up, using our hands to pull ourselves up to the top. This led to a lane which did eventually take us to Helmsdale, arriving at 8.15pm completely worn out!

Helmsdale is a small town with a harbour. We're staying at the Bannockburn Inn in a flat in the annex. We had a lovely meal in the restaurant. We're totally exhausted.

Thursday July 27th

Helmsdale to Dunbeath   **Caithness**   *15 miles*

After yesterday, we decided we'd risk going on the A9. Ian and I wore our high visibility vests. It was not as bad as we feared. It was hard on our feet but mostly there was a verge to step up on when the lorries and coaches came. It was noisy but there were occasional minute silences when nothing came. There were views of the hills and the sea and some trees and wild flowers at the side of the road including ragwort, thrift and sea mayweed.

Progress is much faster by keeping to the main roads and it's cheering when some drivers hoot and wave to support you. But I don't want to keep on the A9. I'd like to try the alternative route again.

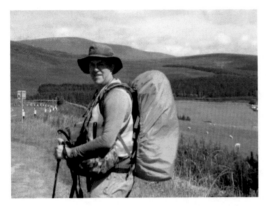

It was a bit midgy when we stopped to rest under some trees. So it's not just the west coast that gets the midges. But this east side is definitely better.

Ian

We're in a nice B & B within a campsite in Dunbeath. Dunbeath is a pleasant village with a harbour. It has one restaurant which was luckily quite nearby and very good. We had a view of the sea from the restaurant and could see

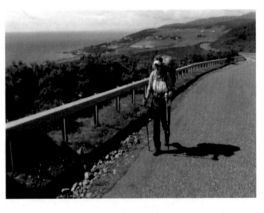

Dunbeath Castle. It's in a most spectacular setting. It's white and on the very edge of the cliff! We were told that a castle has stood there since the 15th century but is mostly 17th century. It's now a family home but it's not open to the public.

Friday July 28th

Dunbeath to Lybster   **Caithness**   *10 miles*

We decided to try Jay Wilson's alternative route once more. However, after climbing one fence where Ian did a Judo roll after falling from it and then a very difficult long stretch of tussocky grass with more fences approaching we decided to go back to the A9.

So we wasted time and energy on that fruitless attempt. The road was OK. There were some small hilly parts. I didn't have much energy today. It must be after that exhausting day on Wednesday. I don't believe that this alternative route of Jay Wilson's will be finished in two years. More like twenty years! We've only seen one stile, no bridges and a few splashes of white paint on walls.

We read that Lybster was once a big herring fishing port but no longer. It is also famous for hosting the "World Championships of Knotty". Knotty is a variant of shinty which is a bit like hockey to the uninitiated.

We looked for a café in Lybster by going half way down a long road through the village to the harbour but there was no café.

The village was a terrible place. It looked like an open prison. We eventually reached a sign pointing to the Antlers which we thought must be a pub. This is where we'd booked in to stay. It was two miles further on from the village. We were shocked to find it was a B & B and therefore we would have nowhere to eat tonight with it not being the pub we'd expected. However, it was great! We were greeted with a pot of tea and chocolate rolls and KitKats. We had a four poster bed and a bath with Radox! And best of all the pleasant owner had a menu for evening meals! We chose steak and chips with strawberries and cream for afters. Sometimes things just turn out fine.

Saturday July 29th

Lybster to Whaligoe   **Caithness**   6 miles

It was a sunny day as we walked along the A99 for most of the way. There were grassy moors and rushes with some heather on the roadside verges. There were hardly any trees. There were some crofts (small farms) and low bungalows. On the verges, there was purple knapweed, yellow lady's bedstraw and red clover. We tried to go back once more to the Jay Wilson alternative route nearer to the cliffs but it was too difficult. The ground was boggy and muddy with no path and we climbed a wall at one place. After a short time, we decided it made our progress too slow and it was too tiring so we returned to the road.

Shortly afterwards, we came to Whaligoe where there was a lane leading to a café and some steps. In fact, we'd found the iconic Whaligoe steps used in Billy Connolly's Tour of Scotland a few years ago on the TV. Whaligoe means "inlet of the whale". We left our big bags outside the café at the top and in beautiful sunshine climbed down the 330 stone steps on a steep zigzag cliff edge route down to the tiny harbour flanked by towering cliffs. In the middle of the 19th century, this was the route the "herring girls" took when they met the fishing boats and unloaded and gutted the fish. They packed them into baskets which they carried

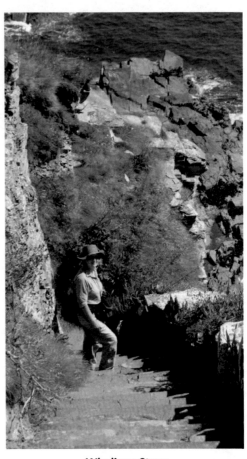

Whaligoe Steps

on their backs and struggled back up to the top. They must have been strong and fit.

Luckily for us, we could go to the café at the top to revive us.

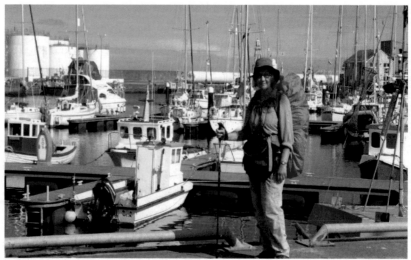

Wick Harbour

Then we caught the bus to Wick so arrived there just after lunch. We are staying in a lovely flat in an old terraced house close to the harbour. There are lots of yachts and boats in the harbour. We were very lucky as we found out that it's the last night of their Gala week in Wick. So tonight we went into the town and saw a wonderful Scottish Pipe and Drum band and watched Scottish dancing in the street.

It was so good. Just what I'd been hoping for. And as we were leaving, we saw a double rainbow over the harbour. A fitting end to a lovely day. One of the best.

Sunday July 30th

Whaligoe to Wick   ***Caithness***   *8 miles*

It was another sunny day today. Ian and I caught a bus back to Whaligoe and walked back to Wick on the A99. There was not so much traffic, probably because it's a Sunday. We passed a sign to a Heritage Museum which we thought we'd go to but it was shut.

On the A99, we met Phil, a very nice Swiss guy who's also walking from Land's End to John O'Groats. He's doing a video of his walk. He's not that young as he's got grey hair but looks very fit. As am I, of course, after walking all this way!

We got to Wick at 1pm. We looked at the boats in the harbour and found it very interesting watching them load up parts of a wind turbine onto very long trailer lorries. The pieces are huge. It was amazing watching the intricate moves the lorry had to make. Then we drifted around a parkland area near the river. We found the shortest street in the world! It's in the Guinness book of records. It's basically just a hotel at a corner and the street name is on the wall of the hotel. I was having my photo taken outside it when we saw Phil again and had a chat. In fact, we went to that hotel this evening for a very tasty meal. The menu was very interesting with unusual and delicious food. We watched Poldark before going to bed.

Monday July 31st

Wick to Keiss **Caithness** *9 miles*

We walked on the A99 in bright sunshine through Wick to Keiss. It was easy walking. Ever since we've left Inverness, I've noticed that lots of houses have statues of animals in their gardens. These are mainly dogs, mostly life size, but some are huge. They are certainly less trouble than the real thing and people tell me it's a safe area so possibly they don't need a real dog to guard them. As we get further north, the land is flatter with fewer trees and more grassy moors.

The pioneers of the Land's End to John O'Groats walk were Robert and John Naylor in 1871. Little did they know it would inspire so many people to do the same. Today we met a man who was going from John O'Groats to Land's End. He was riding a bike and towing a small cart containing his luggage and his dog. Goodness knows how he'll manage on the busy roads! The coaches and lorries are really frightening but at least we can step up onto the verge. The dog will be terrified!

On approaching Keiss, we took a narrow road down to the sandy and pebbly beach. It was lovely. There were wild flowers in abundance: marsh woundwort, sea mayweed and the tall yellow flowers of sow thistle. We sat on some rocks and had a picnic lunch. Keiss is a small fishing village. Keiss has a ruined castle which stands on sheer cliffs overlooking Sinclair's Bay. We're staying in the Sinclair Hotel.

Tuesday August 1st

Keiss to John O'Groats & Duncansby Head **Caithness**   *12 miles*

My last day was a good one. It was sunny and Ian and I walked fast along the main road to John O'Groats. The approach to John O'Groats was beautiful. There was hardly any traffic on the road. The landscape on either side was flat grassy moorland and ahead was the island of Skoma with the hills and mountains of Orkney beyond. The whole scene was bathed in sunshine with a dark curtain of rain moving over the islands from the west. Fortunately, we avoided it. It was very atmospheric and heightened the joy that I was feeling at finishing the challenge.

We got to the B & B at about 1pm to drop the bags off as the actual iconic signpost is further down the road right near the sea. As the proprietor opened the door to us he said. "Have you been down there to the signpost yet? Charles is there." I didn't know what he was talking about and asked who Charles was. "Prince Charles! " With that, we dumped our bags and set off quickly. I just thought it would be a fitting end for Prince Charles to shake my hand as I'd done it for his father's charity — The Duke of Edinburgh's Award Scheme.

When we got there, we saw quite a lot of people near the signpost and a piper was playing. There were some shops and cafes nearby too. I looked at the tourists. Not one was a walker or a cyclist who'd actually done the massive walk or cycle ride. Yet they all went up in turn and had their picture taken by the sign. I felt quite cross thinking they hadn't earned that picture. Eventually, it was my turn and I enjoyed having lots of pictures taken, alone, with Ian and with Squeaky, the mouse puppet who'd done the whole walk with me! Just to show the grandchildren! Prince Charles was nowhere to be

seen. It seems he was in a nearby distillery. His loss! He missed me!

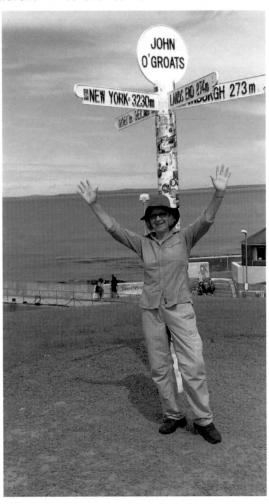

We decided we'd like to walk a bit further...why not...? and go to the actual most easterly point of Scotland which is Duncansby Head. So we walked along the clifftop path to the lighthouse and then even further to look at the massive stacks of Duncansby. These are spectacular huge rocks like pyramids which emerge from a bay.

We walked back and looked at the Inn at John O'Groats which is just near the signpost. This is the reincarnation of the iconic former John O'Groats Hotel which was originally built in 1875. It's white with an octagonal main building with an octagonal tower and has a colourful Norse style extension where all the buildings are painted different bright colours. I could see them as we were walking towards the village and wondered what they were. It was built in 2013.

Just near the Inn is a mound marking the spot where Jan de Groot, a Dutchman, built his famous house in the 15th century. His seven sons quarrelled about who would inherit the most of their father's property. Jan de Groot solved the problem by building an octagonal house with eight doors, one for each of his seven sons and one for himself. Inside was an eight-sided table so that no one occupied the head of the table.

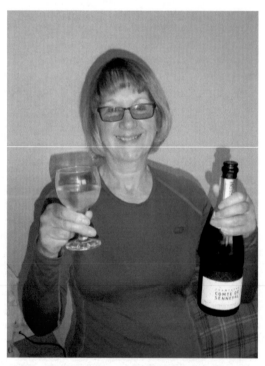

Jan de Groot ran a ferry to Orkney and charged 2p a trip. The coin became known as a "groat". This is why eventually his name was changed to John O'Groats. And thus the actual place took on the name.

We saw a ferry crowded with people going across to Orkney and we wished we'd thought ahead and left enough time to make the trip. I'd really like to explore the islands but it'll have to wait for another time. Such a pity when we're so close now. But Ian has used up all his holidays till next April by coming to join me so much on this adventure.

We celebrated in a restaurant with a lovely meal and I emailed and texted all my family and friends. On returning to our B & B, I was amazed to find cards and parcels for me. I didn't know anyone knew where I would be staying.

There was a bottle of champagne from my walking group and chocolates too and a big card from them with messages from them all. Marvellous! Patsy sent me a card and chocolates and Mike and Lorraine sent me a trophy and chocolates. Zoë and the boys sent me good wishes and the boys had written me a card with a picture of them at the signpost at Land's End! I'm glad they now know where I started from. They'd also made me a big medal reading "Well done Gran!" Wonderful! The Cleethorpes Chronicle rang up and I gave a last interview with them about my adventure.

What next?

I found it hard to settle when I got back. Every night for the first two or three weeks, I would dream I was walking in Scotland and on the moments before waking I would think "where am I and where am I going today?"

People ask what next? I certainly don't fancy doing another ridiculously long walk. It was too hard, too much of a slog. There were moments of enjoyment, especially when I had friends or family with me but mostly it was just hours and hours of walking. It would have been better without having to carry a heavy rucksack.

So what next? Coming from Lincolnshire, I've never been any good at hills. However, after walking the length of Britain which is actually full of hills, I've got pretty good at them. So I'm thinking about climbing hills and mountains as my next challenge. I think I'll start with the three Yorkshire Peaks, Pen-y-ghent, Whernside and Ingleborough (but not all at once) and if they are not too awful, I may go on to attempt the three national peaks of Scafell Pike, Snowdon and Ben Nevis. There's no rush. I shall climb them slowly and hopefully enjoy the views going up and down. After all, I'm only going to be 70 this year so lots of time!

The main thing is I think everyone needs a challenge. A reason to get up in the morning. It's good to have something to aspire to and a goal to work towards. That's why I wanted to encourage young people to face a challenge and walk in the hills and climb mountains. By doing my walk, I raised £3000 for the disadvantaged youngsters of North East Lincolnshire who struggle to pay for the trips and activities in the Duke of Edinburgh's Award Scheme. Part of the proceeds of this book will go towards that charity. So thanks for buying a copy.

January 2018

During the summer of 2018 I filled in the miles that I had to miss out, due mostly to bad weather. These are:

6 miles from Carrbrook to Standedge

4 miles of the Lowther Hills to Wanlockhead.

13 miles from Abington to Lesmahagow

See Appendix on the next page.

I also climbed Pen y Ghent and Ingleborough with Ian. I climbed Snowdon on my own and Scafell Pyke with my daughter Zoë.

Appendix

Walks missed out in 2017 that have now been done.

Saturday May 12th 2018

Carrbrook to Standedge   **West Yorkshire**   6 miles

The Pennine Bridleway

What a change from last year when I was so down and exhausted and the weather was dull, dismal and rainy! (Page79 and 80).

Today it was fine sunny weather, perfect for walking and I felt fit. This time Ian accompanied me. The tracks were good and never went into any fields though the route went through farmland with cows, sheep and lambs on the other side of fences. It went through lovely bluebell woods too. Despite being on the eastern edge of Manchester the Pennine Bridleway was delightful. It was well signed and there were wonderful views of the hills and moors. We had lunch at a hotel in Diggle sitting outside enjoying the views of the hills.

Monday August 6th 2018

Wanlockhead to where we got to last year and back   8 miles

Dumfries and Galloway

Last year, in terrible weather, we were blown down in the Lowther hills while attempting to reach Wanlockhead and had to hitch a lift to our accommodation. (See page 108).
So this year we decided to start at Wanlockhead and walk in reverse to what we did last year. We had to go there and back as there was no other way of getting back to our car. We decided to follow a different path from the Southern Upland Way to start with. This was marked as a private road belonging to the Radar station but we

didn't think that applied to walkers. It was an easy tarmac road leading gently upwards to the Lowther Hill Radar station. Heather and bilberries were growing on the moorland and we saw a few sheep. The weather started misty and cool and quickly developed into thick fog with visibility down to 30 yards. However there was no wind. Suddenly the huge tower of the radar station loomed out of the mist. We had our lunch under the shelter of its spherical shield.

After that we started walking on the grassy moors. Luckily it was not as boggy as before due to the long spell of dry weather everyone has had. We followed vague tracks across the moors following posts looming out of the fog from time to time. There were some level parts but more long drags of hills up and down. After three and a half hours we reached the point where we'd had to give up due to the gales and mist. We had our lunch and sat on a gate for a picture then turned round for the long plod back. It was eerily quiet. We heard no birds, saw no one and even the sheep had disappeared. However we found a metal hut near to the radar station to have a nice break in. On the long road back down to Wanlockhead we were rewarded by the mist starting to clear revealing the most marvellous views of hills and reservoirs with some mist hanging between the hills.

Tuesday August 7th 2018

Abingdon to Lesmahago   **Lanarkshire**   17 miles

Last year I had had enough of wild camping and so we decided to try to find a B & B instead. The only one we could find was further on so that's why I missed out part of the journey of LeJog. (Page 109 & 110)

Ian and I set off from Abington Services which was where we got the bus from last year to Lesmahagow. We walked along a quiet "B" road and to our delight found a lovely cycle path to walk on away from the road. There were wild flower verges of purple tufted vetch, white ox-eye daisies, the lovely deep purple sheep's-bit scabious and yellow bird's foot trefoil. There were lots of tall pink spikes of rose-bay willow herb in full bloom.

We saw one of my favourite signs advertising a Hotel Truck Stop which to me meant a cup of hot frothy coffee. Unfortunately when we got there it was closed.

Along the way we met Jim Thompson who we discovered was doing LeJog on a scooter! Not a motorised one but an adult sized push scooter. Is this a first? Amazing! He told us he does change feet as he scoots along to equalise the pressure on his feet. He's doing it from John O'Groats to Land's End in one month. He was travelling very light, just a couple of plastic bags tied to his handlebars. He sleeps in a bivvy bag on the roadsides mostly but last night he was exhausted and a farmer let him sleep in a barn. I asked him if there were any mice or rats in the barn and he replied that he didn't know as he was fast asleep. His feet must hurt as he can only go on tarmac not the soft grass of field tracks and footpaths that walkers can use. I gave him a donation to his charity.

After six miles we had to walk along the edge of the noisy "B" road for a couple of miles. Then we turned off onto a narrow road through a pleasant wood. We had our lunch here and lay in the sun for a pleasant rest. We turned onto a track through woodland. However the track soon disappeared and the going got more difficult with long grass. Then we found a long track by forests and past a wind farm. There was heather and wild flowers in abundance especially lots of white sneezewort flowers! These are quite rare in Lincolnshire. We saw and heard a buzzard and watched a pair of them soaring and calling over the trees.

We went over a bridge to a field of cows and bullocks which moved away leaving a solitary bull looking at us. We stayed on the bridge till it eventually followed the cattle. We tentatively edged our way over the bridge keeping one eye on the bull who kept his eye on us as he paused to keep looking back at us. We made it to the gate before he changed his mind and came after us.

There were more cattle in the next field, very fine looking beasts, all different colours. They ran towards us to have a look and then ran away from us again thankfully. A beautiful white horse looked over the fence at us so we fed him some long grass.

Eventually after many hours we arrived at the small town of Lesmahagow. We walked around the streets for ages till we discovered where the correct bus stop was. We found we'd missed the 7pm bus and the next one didn't go till 9pm. So we went in a pub for a well-deserved drink and got chatting to the locals. They were so welcoming and cheery that we couldn't get away to go and find a pub that had food as we discovered that this one only served drinks. It was very entertaining talking to them though I couldn't understand half of what they were saying as their Scottish accents were so broad. Ian could though and it seems we were getting a potted history of the town, ghost stories and all.

We caught the bus back after some fish and chips. We nearly didn't get off at Abington as the driver had forgotten we were on the bus and almost didn't stop! We had a hot chocolate before collapsing after doing 17 miles!

Clothes and Equipment

Summer jacket Karrimor. Not waterproof replaced with Rohan winter jacket, waterproof.	Sponge-bag
	First-aid bag
Lightweight showerproof jacket.	Mat to sit on
Neck warmer	Torch & camera
Overtrousers, Rohan	High visibility vest
Trousers, Craghoppers	Survival bag
Lightweight trousers	Compass & binoculars
T shirts short- sleeved x2 Regatta	Maps and map case
Long sleeved shirt, Peter Storm	Whistle
Fleece jumper x2	Water bottles x2
Lightweight evening top x2	Boot wax
Lightweight shoes & Slipper socks	Notebook and pens and pencils
Waterproof socks x2	Glasses x2
Evening socks x2	Credit and Debit card
Walking socks x2	Cash
Underwear x2	Mobile phone
Thermal long sleeved vests x2	2 carbon walking poles
Nightie & Thermal Long Johns	Backpack (Lowe Alpine 75 L capacity)
Warm gloves	Small Daypack
Waterproof gloves	Bum bag
Liner gloves	Leather waterproof boots Meindl Size 5 replaced with Grisport boots Size 6 not waterproof despite label stating they are.
Gaiters & waterproof hat	
Warm hat, sunhat & peak cap	

Mileage totals

Mileage		Walking days	Average miles per day	Days off
Stage 1	282	25	11.1	3
Stage 2	255	22	11.6	1
Stage 3	211	18	12	1
Stage 4	246	20	12.3	0
Stage 5	82	8	10.2	0
Stage 6	149	13	11.6	o
Total	1225	106	11.5	5

Long Distance Paths

The Camel Trail	1 day
The Two Castles Trail	1 day
The Two Moors Way	1 day
The Cotswold Way	9 days
The Heart of England Way	7 days
The Staffordshire Way	1 day
The Limestone Way	1 day
The Trans Pennine Trail	1 days
Pennine Bridleway	4 days
The Pennine Way	5 days
The Ribble Way	1 day
The Dales Way	5 days
The Cumbria Way	6 days
The Annandale Way	1 day
The West Highland Way	8 days
The Great Glen Way	8 days

County	Local Delicacy
Cornwall	Cornish pasty
Devon	Devon cream tea
Somerset	Cider
Gloucestershire	Double Gloucester cheese
Warwickshire	Warwickshire Truckle (cheese)
Staffordshire	Oatcake
Derbyshire	Bakewell Tart
Yorkshire	Parkin
Lancashire	Hotpot
Cumbria	Sticky toffee pudding
Dumfries and Galloway	Ecclefechan tart
Lanarkshire	Porridge
Dunbartonshire	Raspberries
Stirlingshire	Haggis, neeps and tatties
Perthshire	Venison
Argyll	Shortbread
Inverness-shire	Cranachan
Ross-shire	Scottish Tablet
Sutherland	Salmon
Caithness	Tattie scones

Success is to be measured not so much by the position one has reached in life, as by the obstacles which one has overcome while trying to succeed.

Booker T. Washington